MW00813076

ROYAL INBREEDING
AND
OTHER MALADIES

'In this Kingdom, as is well known, a King is constituted not by the wishes of the people or by election or the right of war but by the propagation of blood.'

Margaret of Burgundy

ROYAL INBREEDING
AND
OTHER MALADIES

A History of Royal Intermarriage and Its Consequences

JULIANA CUMMINGS

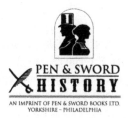

PEN & SWORD
HISTORY

AN IMPRINT OF PEN & SWORD BOOKS LTD.
YORKSHIRE - PHILADELPHIA

First published in Great Britain in 2024 by
PEN AND SWORD HISTORY
An imprint of
Pen & Sword Books Ltd
Yorkshire – Philadelphia

ISBN 978 1 39901 219 5

A CIP catalogue record for this book is available from the British Library.

Typeset in Times New Roman 12/16 by
SJmagic DESIGN SERVICES, India.
Printed and bound in the UK by CPI Group (UK) Ltd.

Pen & Sword Books Limited incorporates the imprints of Atlas, Archaeology,
Aviation, Discovery, Family History, Fiction, History, Maritime, Military,
After the Battle, Military Classics, Politics, Select, Transport, True Crime,
Air World, Frontline Publishing, Leo Cooper, Remember When,
Seaforth Publishing, The Praetorian Press, Wharncliffe Local History,
Wharncliffe Transport, Wharncliffe True Crime and White Owl.

For a complete list of Pen & Sword titles please contact
PEN & SWORD BOOKS LIMITED
George House, Units 12 & 13, Beevor Street, Off Pontefract Road,
Barnsley, South Yorkshire, S71 1HN, England
E-mail: enquiries@pen-and-sword.co.uk
Website: www.pen-and-sword.co.uk

or

PEN AND SWORD BOOKS
1950 Lawrence Rd, Havertown, PA 19083, USA
E-mail: uspen-and-sword@casematepublishers.com
Website: www.penandswordbooks.com

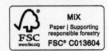

Contents

Introduction

On 9 October 1646, King Philip IV of Spain received word that Balthasar Charles, his only son, had died of smallpox after receiving his last sacrament. He was 16 years old and the king's only hope of carrying on the Habsburg dynasty. Philip had also lost his wife, Elisabeth of France, only two years prior.

The king was utterly devastated by the loss of his son, to whom he had been a good father. But what plagued him the most was the possibility of strengthening Spain's relationship with the Austrian Habsburgs may be over. Philip had no choice but to take another wife.

In 1649, at the age of 44, King Philip IV married 14-year-old Mariana of Austria, who had been betrothed to Balthasar Charles before he died. Mariana was the daughter of Ferdinand III, Holy Roman Emperor.

She was also King Philip's niece.

Two years later, the new queen of Spain gave birth to the first of five children; only two would survive to adulthood. On 6 November 1661, Mariana would deliver the future King Charles II of Spain, who would become the most inbred European royal in history. Of the fifty-six ancestors of the new heir's mother, forty-eight of them were also the ancestors of his father.

Perhaps Mariana knew something was amiss right away. While her labour had been relatively easy, the child that lay in her arms was clearly not the child described in the birth announcement. The official gazette said the future king was: 'Most beautiful in features, with a large head and dark skin and somewhat plump.'

The child instead had a deformity on one ear with sores on his neck. He was also considerably weak and sickly looking. Nonetheless, he was the heir to the Habsburg dynasty. He would also cause its end due to his failure to govern the nation and, most importantly, father a successor.

Charles II of Spain would grow into an adult who had control of Spain's future, despite his inability to rule. His jaw was deformed to the point where he could not chew his food correctly or speak coherently. He drooled constantly and spent his life in considerable pain. His intellectual abilities were subpar at best, and he had no understanding of how to bed either of his two wives.

Like many monarchies throughout Europe and the rest of the world, providing an heir to the throne came at all costs. With no knowledge of genetics or modern science, royals would continue to interbreed with blood relatives with the notion that they would preserve the bloodline. There existed no understanding of why stillbirths or mental illness occurred, decade after decade. A monarch's most important job would be to see that their dynasty continued.

The history of the Western world shows an intricate tangle of royal families who passed brides around like trading cards to secure alliances with foreign countries. The fairy tales of the handsome king and beautiful queen living happily in a luxurious castle were, more often than not, just that: fairy tales. Brides especially had no choice in the matter of their marriages, and little consideration was taken into age, appearance, or personality. Girls, sometimes as young as 10 or 11 years old, were often sent to neighbouring countries where they did not speak the language and had no understanding of court etiquette. The main objective was to procreate, whether with a non-relative, a cousin, or an uncle.

Many royals overlooked canon law on consanguinity, which prohibited anyone more closely related than seventh cousins from marriage, or were granted a dispensation in order to marry within the family.

Even for royals that may not have been inbred, there was also the possibility of inheriting a debilitating genetic disorder that would be passed through generations without knowing why or how to end it.

While Queen Victoria was one of the most successful monarchs of the United Kingdom, her genes carried a disease that would all but destroy the Russian Monarchy.

While the illusion of the monarchy is often looked upon with awe, there lies a truth behind the crown that is hard for us to understand today.

I have always had a fascination with the health of monarchs throughout history. And through years of research, I have come to learn that the majority of disorders suffered by royals were perfectly preventable if there had been an understanding of genetics. While it may have been hundreds of years ago, it is important to remember that these people are not just paintings or photographs in a history book. These people were real, and they lived and breathed as we do now. Only they had little choice in their future and often lived a very painful existence that seems unimaginable to us today.

I've done my best to pull back the layers of history and discover more about the men and women who ruled dynasties despite their mental and physical inabilities. They shaped history, for good or for bad, and deserve to be better understood.

These are their stories.

Acknowledgements

I want to thank everyone who has continued to support me through my writing career: my husband, parents, and family. Thanks to my friends, Jane, Brenda, and Kristen, who have always been there to egg me on. You are the best.

I want to thank everyone at Pen & Sword, who have been nothing but amazing. Thank you so much for your patience!

I also want to acknowledge the past members of royalty who have suffered from disorders none of us can comprehend. Through no fault of their own, they were born into a family that expected so much more of them than they were able to give.

Chapter One

A History of Genetics and What Happens When It Goes Wrong

To dive into the spider's web of royal marriage and intermarriage, we must start at the beginning. Understanding the history of heredity and genetic dispositions is essential if we want to grasp the foundation of what was going on in the marriage bed of royals, and why. What is it that makes us what and who we are? And how? Are we guaranteed disaster if we trifle with the gene pool?

The history of understanding genetics dates to the classical era. The most influential ideas on heredity stem from Hippocrates (460-370 BC) and Aristotle (384-322 BC). During the fifth century BC, Hippocrates had a theory on genetics known as the 'bricks and mortar' theory. This theory being that the materials that made up genetics were physical substances that came from certain parts of the body, almost like an invisible seed. Hippocrates focused specifically on the idea that all parts of the body stemmed from the male's semen. These building blocks were transmitted during sexual intercourse, where they reconstructed themselves in the mother's womb to develop into a baby.

Hippocrates was also of the understanding that one's physical characteristics were acquired or inherited. For example, one who may have had strong biceps, had 'strong bicep parts' and would have passed this to his offspring, ensuring that the child would also have strong biceps.

It was quite some time later that Aristotle would sharply criticise the beliefs of Hippocrates. He believed that if one were physically handicapped or had become disfigured, they could still have a

1

physically normal child. He also thought that a parent could pass on traits that may not have been shown at a young age. For example, one who went grey quickly could pass this on to their children, who would not reveal their own grey hair until later in life.

Aristotle also objected to Hippocrates' bricks-and-mortar theory because he felt heredity involved a transmission of information. His theory was known as the 'blueprint model' and is still referred to today.

Aristotle also stressed the importance of blood as part of heredity. He believed that it was the blood that provided the materials needed to build all aspects of the human body and could be passed from generation to generation. He specified that the semen from a male was cleansed blood and that a woman's menstrual blood was the equivalent of semen. He felt that a baby would be produced when these two materials came together in the womb during intercourse. He thought that the blood contained the essence of heredity, and the baby would develop from the influence of this essence.

We often hear people today referring to hereditary traits in the blood, and royals were obsessed with keeping the bloodlines of a family in order to preserve a monarchy. We now know that there was some truth to Aristotle's theory, but it wouldn't be understood for years to come.

Under the influence of philosophies developed by Epicurus of Athens (341–270 BC), scholars in the Hellenistic and Roman eras were led to ideas proven as scientific fact today. During the fifth century BC, Democritus of Abdera (460–370 BC) discovered the building blocks of matter, calling them *atomos,* known as atoms today. According to Democritus, atomos were solid and indestructible and existed not only for building matter, but also for the qualities of the human soul.

Epicurus took Democritus' ideas on atomic physics and the theory of Aristotle and combined them. He suggested that these atomos are constantly connected, forming the molecules which would produce all living organisms. While Aristotle was under the belief that it was only men who contributed to heredity, Epicurus felt that it was both men and women who played a part. And he believed they did so equally. It is also thought that it was Epicurus who described dominant, recessive, and co-dominant inheritance.

Theories of genetics and heredity would change throughout the Middle Ages and through the middle of the Victorian period. Still, modern genetics and the principles of inheritance were not truly understood until 1865, when the ideas of Gregor Mendel (1822–1884) were proposed.

Gregor Mendel was a meteorologist, biologist, and mathematician. He was also an Augustinian Frair at St Thomas Abbey in Margraviate of Moravia, the present-day Czech Republic.

While studying at the University of Vienna, Mendel devoted much of his time to physics and mathematics. He also took a liking to study the anatomy and physiology of plants. While experimenting with different pea plants, he established the rules of heredity, known as *The Laws of Mendelian Inheritance*.

Mendel discovered several characteristics of pea plants: height, pod shape and colour, flower position and colour, and seed shape and colour. He showed that when a yellow pea and a green pea were cross-bred, the result was always yellow seeds. However, in the following generation, the green peas reappeared at a ratio of one green to three yellow. Mendel called this 'recessive' and 'dominant' regarding the traits of the plant.

In 1866, Mendel published his works explaining these 'invisible factors', as he called them. These factors determine the trait of an organism, and today, these factors are known as genes.

At the time, Mendel's work wasn't given much consideration, as most conversations about heredity focused on Charles Darwin's (1809–1882) theory of evolution by natural selection. Darwin's theory says that organisms produce more offspring than can survive in the environment. Those better equipped would grow to maturity and reproduce themselves, and those not well equipped would perish.

It was in 1868 that Charles Darwin proposed his pangenesis theory. His theory described the components of inheritance between parents and children and how those components would affect the child's development. It was Darwin that came up with the concept of gemmules, a mass of cells that can develop into a new organism. Darwin felt that the environment surrounding an organism could alter the gemmules, causing them to congregate in the parents' reproductive organs and then be passed to offspring. Darwin's' theory eventually lost popularity as biologists replaced his theory with germ plasm theory and chromosomal theories of inheritance.

What is interesting in Darwin's case is that his studies of heredity included experiments on the effects of inbreeding in plants and animals. He found the results were often weaker and more sickly offspring. So, we can assume that he understood somewhat how inbreeding could affect progeny. And yet, he still married into his own family.

When Darwin was 29, he proposed to his first cousin, Emma Wedgewood (1808–1896). He must have wondered if his close relation to his wife had something to do with the fact that the health of his children was not great. In a letter to a friend, Darwin refers to the health of his children and says of them, 'they are not very robust'.

Any concerns Darwin had about his offspring would have been valid, as an analysis published by Tim Berra, Professor Emeritus at Ohio State University in Mansfield, found a considerable amount of inbreeding in Darwin's family. Aside from his marriage to his cousin, the family had other instances of close relative matches. There was also a significant association between inbreeding and child mortality in his family history.

Four generations of the Darwins and Wedgewoods were studied and found to have a higher-than-average child death rate than that of the general public. There was also a reduction in their physical fitness, which may have been what Darwin was referring to when he said his children were 'not very robust'.

None of Darwin's children had any obvious deformities, but three of his children did die from an infectious disease. Infectious disease is more likely in inbred children due to a weakened immune system.

His first daughter, Annie (1841–1851), died of tuberculosis at the age of 10, and another daughter, Mary (1842), only lived for twenty-three days. Darwin's last child, a boy named Charles (1856–1858), was born with Down Syndrome, but it was scarlet fever that would take his life at just 18 months old.

In 1897, Dutch Botanist Hugo de Vries (1848–1935) published his own works on genetics after reading some of Mendel's previous papers. De Vries believed each trait of a human being was governed by two particles of information, one from each parent. Two other botanists, Carl Correns (1864–1933) and Erich Von Tschermak (1871–1962), also referred to Mendel's papers for their work. And by 1915, the basic principles of Mendelian genetics were being studied, leading to acceptance in 1925.

By the 1940s and 1950s, biologists were able to study and understand gene theory and that it was DNA that held these genes, leading up to what we know today, that we, as humans, each have forty-six chromosomes, twenty-three from each parent.

Each chromosome holds a genetic code that determines everything from eye colour to intelligence to blood type. But what happens when a child inherits a defective gene? Inherited characteristics can be traced to one particular gene or the interaction of several genes. Many inherited factors not associated with gender are still carried on the sex chromosomes. This is the case with haemophilia, the disorder that would plague the family of Queen Victoria of England (1819–1901) and generations to follow.

In the case of haemophilia, it is understood now that the defect causing the disorder was with the X chromosome, which is why women can be carriers but will never suffer from the disease. If a woman gave birth to a boy, he may inherit her defective gene and manifest the disease. If the same woman were to give birth to a girl, she may inherit the gene but only be a carrier. One of the unfortunate aspects of haemophilia is that girls who inherit the gene often do not know they are carriers and can go on to have unaffected sons. Victoria's family is a classic example of how the inheritance of haemophilia works. Two of the queen's daughters, who were carriers of the gene, passed it to their sons, who, in turn, became affected. But this same gene that was also passed down to daughters only made those daughters new carriers of the trait.

Autosomal dominant inheritance is when offspring get a normal gene from one parent and a defective gene from the other. This child now has a 50 per cent chance of getting the disorder. Autosomal recessive inheritance is when both parents carry and pass on a faulty gene to their child. This child now has a 25 per cent chance of inheriting both copies of the defective gene and a 50 per cent chance of inheriting the gene and passing it on to their children. And throughout most of Ancient and European history, the inheritance of genes was not considered or even understood.

The statistics are based on the assumption that both parents stem from families that are not related. But what happens when a child's parents are related, as was very common throughout history, especially when it came to royalty? In the case of parents being blood relatives, chances of inheriting defective genes increase even more, and are often the beginning of a downward spiral in reproduction.

Inbreeding increases homozygosity, or alleles, which are two or more versions of a gene, leading to decreased ability to survive reproduction. One who inherits these alleles is often referred to as inbred.

Inbreeding or reproduction between blood relatives is a practice that is considered taboo throughout the world. But that wasn't always the case. And it's sometimes used in the animal kingdom. Selective breeding is sometimes used in breeding livestock to produce a new and desirable trait, and it can also be used in cases where a recessive gene is hoped to be bred out. It's also not uncommon for several insects to inbreed.

Aside from the historical prevalence of nobility, inbreeding is especially problematic in small, uneducated populations, but there are cases where it is done by choice. This is usually dependent on culture and religion.

Middle Eastern and African territories show the highest frequency of consanguinity. The link between inbreeding and Islam may be due to the widening Islamic populations. Many Islamic populaces have historically participated in close family relations. Several disorders have arisen from prevalent inbreeding in Egypt, Lebanon, Saudi Arabia, and Israel. Children are sometimes born with congenital heart defects or malformations, neural tube defects, and hydrocephalus. Cleft palates also show up in children in Palestine and Lebanon. In Qatar, there is a higher rate of close family relations, which has increased genetic diseases such as hearing loss.

Relations between first cousins double the risk of infant death and mental and physical disabilities. The closer the relationship of the parents, and the more generations of inbreeding that have occurred, the more problems can pile up and produce children with multiple defects.

Historically, until there was an understanding of how genetics worked, people didn't realise that inbreeding caused problems. Now, however, we have an excellent understanding of things, which explains why the practice has decreased considerably over time.

However, what I found surprising in my research for this book is that current day inbreeding in the Western world was not as rare as I thought. While it is severely frowned upon in the United States, the practice isn't illegal in all fifty states. It is legal to marry a first cousin in nineteen US states. Two per cent of marriages in the United States are between second or first cousins. This practice is more prevalent in rural areas of the country, in states such as North Carolina, West Virginia and Kentucky. Roughly 70 per cent of the families practising inbreeding are in hugely desolate areas.

In eastern Kentucky, the percentage of inbred families is higher than in the rest of the state, in part due to the ruralness of the Appalachian Mountains. Families often settle there due to the low cost of living and choose not to leave. Because many of these areas have very little interaction with others, it is not uncommon for families to procreate with one another.

In 1830, a Frenchman named Martin Fugate settled in an area known as Troublesome Creek in eastern Kentucky and married a woman named Elizabeth Smith. What Martin and Elizabeth didn't know was that they both carried a recessive gene that led to four of their children being born with skin that had a striking blue colour.

The family lived where there were no roads, and it wouldn't be until 1910 that railroads reached that part of Kentucky. Due to this, the Fugate children intermarried. Zachariah, the son of Martin and Elizabeth, married his mother's sister. Over the next hundred years, the Fugate family continued to live in isolation. Their repeated inbreeding allowed for the continuation of the recessive gene that eventually got the family their nickname: the Blue Fugates.

It wasn't until 1960 that two members of the Fugate family reached out to the University of Kentucky in the hopes of understanding their condition. Doctors determined they carried a very rare gene for a hereditary blood disorder that caused high levels of methaemoglobin, a blue version of healthy haemoglobin, in their blood. It was because of the family's isolation and inbreeding that this incredibly rare disorder was so pronounced in their bloodline.

As recently as 2020, a gentleman named Mark Laita has been filming documentaries about a similar family who lives in southwestern West Virginia. The Whitaker Family is believed to suffer from reduced cognitive abilities that stem from inbreeding. While living together in a run-down home with dirt floors in a desolate part of the state, most of the family members are non-verbal or have obvious facial deformities. While a few family members appear somewhat intelligent, others communicate by grunting and making barking noises. However, like many other families, the Whitakers are happy and take pride in caring for each other, despite their intellectual disabilities.

Today we are better prepared to study and understand the effect inbreeding has on offspring. And the list is lengthy. Inbred children who survive into child-rearing age have been known to show a decrease in fertility due to a problem with sperm transport, ovulation, and fertilisation.

The Hutterites, members of a religious sect known as the anabaptists, are believed to practice intermarriage. The group lives in communal areas throughout the Northern United States and Canada, and marriage outside their group is prohibited.

The rare genetic disorder, Bowen Hutterite Syndrome, has been found predominately in this group of people. Growth delays during infancy are common, along with malformations of the face and head, which give those with the disorder a distinctive appearance. Restricted movement in the fingers is noted, as well as foot deformities. Bowen Hutterite Syndrome is an inherited autosomal recessive trait.

Retinitis Pigmentosa, a term given to inherited retinal disorders, which cause poor vision and blindness, has been noted in families living in rural Kentucky, parts of southwest England, and Australia.

In the Adirondack Mountains in New York State, a small mountain ridge known as the Hollow is home to a family that has practised inbreeding for almost 200 years. Two farming families, the Allens and Kathans, settled in the area in the early nineteenth century. The area possessed no local officials, and authorities didn't intervene with the family. Economic hard times of the 1930s forced many families from the mountains, except the Allens, who chose to stay.

By the 1960s, most of the descendants of the original family isolated themselves. They lived in run-down homes and trailers with dirt floors but had no desire to leave the area.

During the making of a 1975 documentary about the family, it was discovered that there were roughly 200 intermarried blood relatives throughout the years. It was clear by speaking with family members that they were perfectly happy staying where they were. The documentary sparked the intervention of social workers, but the help was turned away.

The case with these isolated instances seems to have one thing in common – these actions do not appear to be done with malice. These people are often uneducated and set in their ways. Because of their isolation, they know no other way of life.

One of the more disturbing stories of modern-day intermarriage comes from Australia. The Colt family from New South Wales originally started in 1948 with a woman named June, and has a long and troublesome history of inbreeding. In 1966, June married a man named Timothy Colt, and they relocated to Australia from New Zealand. June, who came from parents who were related, and Timothy had seven children of their own.

Over the next several decades, the family produced twenty-five children and grandchildren, who have continued to survive on a remote farm, living in tents and run-down shacks. Reports state that their living conditions are filthy and dangerous. The matriarch, Betty Colt, and the patriarch, Charlie Colt, were brought to justice in 2012, but not before severe damage was done. Both Betty and Charlie had sexual relationships with their family with the full knowledge of what they were doing. Betty had relations with at least two of her sons, producing thirteen children. Mothers and daughters shared the same father, girls were raped by uncles and brothers, and the lineage continued with more incestual relations between mothers and sons. At least one of the children died from Zellweger Syndrome, which is associated with incest and causes certain brain disorders, as well as problems with the kidneys and liver; it has a high infant-mortality rate. The family shared decades of living with no personal hygiene, grade school-like education, hearing loss, gum and tooth decay, and illiteracy.

Whether it is a consensual relationship or not, it is clear that intermarriage still exists today, and the results are disastrous. Understanding and studying these people can give us a greater idea of what some of the most inbred royal families must have been like throughout history. Many royals, while not necessarily inbred, have also passed down devastating genetic defects of which they were more than likely unaware. While each dynasty may have had different formalities, they all had one thing in common: intermarriage was intentional.

Chapter Two

The Monarchy and
Why It Was so Important

Until the twentieth century, monarchies were the world's most common form of government. They were slowly phased out over time, but forty-three nations still have a monarchy today. Most modern monarchies tend to function as part of legal and ceremonial roles but have little or no political power. Ever since the first known monarchy was established, however, carrying on a dynasty was the main objective for many nations.

Traditionally, a monarchy is a system of government in which the head of state, or monarch, is appointed for life. In rare cases, abdication may cause an early succession. In Britain, absolute monarchies emerged after the social turmoil of the Black Death, leading monarchs to create a centralised state. The British constitutional monarchy was established in 1688 following the Glorious Revolution after the deposition of James II of England and VII of Scotland. In an absolute monarchy, the monarch is the sole ruler, and in a constitutional monarchy, the monarch's powers are outlined in a constitution.

The monarchy is the most ancient of political systems, and almost every country on earth has been ruled by a monarch at one time or another. In an absolute monarchy, the power vested in that one person is usually through the inheritance of the eldest son. In European and Ancient history, a powerful monarch was one that held society together and was the connection to the divine.

The idea of the monarchy originated in prehistoric times, and one of the first documented monarchs was Narmer of Egypt (3273–2987 BC). Narmer, who lived during the Early Dynastic Period, was an Egyptian

Pharaoh considered the founder of the First Dynasty and king of Unified Egypt.

While European kings and queens believed they were God's representatives on earth, the Ancient Egyptians believed themselves to be actual gods. The Pharaoh was one of the oldest ruling monarchs in history, and they had absolute authority in Egypt. Aside from being a living god, the Pharaoh was the head of the political system and was responsible for the economy and for the good of his people. The Pharaoh was the central figure in Ancient Egypt, and if he didn't keep the gods happy, it was believed they could withhold their blessings of well-being over the people, which could lead to famine, disease, and other suffering.

During Narmer's time, Egypt was divided into upper and lower sections. Upper Egypt was more urbanised, while lower Egypt relied more on agriculture. The city of Nagada was a rival power base between the two, and Narmer wanted to overcome the city. By doing so, he would have unified Egypt, paving the way for total affinity.

Narmer married Princess Neithhotep of Nagada to strengthen the two lands. Using his military skills and prowess, Narmer led expeditions through lower Egypt and expanded his territory into Canaan and Nubia. He initiated large building projects and established urbanization.

King Namer had established a dynasty that would be the foundation of Egypt for years to come. He was believed to have been succeeded by his son, Hor-Aha, the second Pharaoh of the First Dynasty. Most Egyptologists agree that his reign was lengthy. Djer (3040 BC), the son of Hor-Aha, ruled as the third Pharoah of the First Dynasty for forty-one years. Djer was succeeded by his wife, who served as Queen Consort to his son, Den (2970 BC). Egypt's First Dynasty ruled for about 200 years.

Until the Fourth Dynasty in 2550 BC, Pharoahs had the greatest power, but this gradually waned over time and Ancient Egypt finally lost its power to the Romans in 30 BC. In the tenth century BC, nomadic Libyans gradually took over seats of power and in the eighth century BC, the Kushites claimed the Egyptian throne, which let to the ultimate downfall of the Pharoah.

The Success of Eleanor of Aquitaine

European monarchies in the early Middle Ages were more like a collection of small areas ruled by Lords under the feudal system. This system allowed the monarch to reap all the benefits as they ruled over the entire kingdom, claiming they had the divine right to govern.

Eleanor of Aquitaine (1122–1204) stands out as one of the Middle Ages' most effective and influential rulers. Aside from being queen of France and England and preserving chivalry at court, she also led a crusade to the Holy Land.

Born in what is southern France today in either 1122 or 1123, Eleanor was educated by her father, William X, Duke of Aquitaine (1098–1137). Her studies included philosophy, literature, and language. At the age of 5, she became her father's heir.

Eleanor spent much of her early teen years as an active woman who loved horseback riding. She was only 15 when her father passed away, and she immediately became the Duchess of Aquitaine, along with becoming the most desirable single woman in all of Europe.

Placed under the guardianship of Louis VI (1081–1137), king of France, she was betrothed to his son and heir, Louis VII (1120–1180) in April of 1137. She and Louis were married in July 1137. King Louis VI died the next month from dysentery, and on Christmas Day of the same year, Louis VII and Eleanor were crowned the new king and queen of France.

Because Louis VII was young, inexperienced, and arrogant, he made several diplomatic and military mistakes that put him at odds against several powerful nobles, as well as Pope Innocent II (1143). But when Pope Eugene III (1088–1153) called for a crusade in 1145, Louis eagerly responded. Eleanor joined her husband on the dangerous journey west. The turbulence of the crusade caused the couple to become increasingly alienated from one another, forcing Eleanor to seek an annulment of the marriage. The Council of Beaugency declared that Louis and Eleanor were too closely related for their marriage to be legal and an annulment was granted in March of 1152 and their two daughters were left in the king's custody.

Eleanor married Henry Plantagenet, Count of Anjou and Duke of Normandy (1133–1189) in May of 1152, and within two years, they were crowned king and queen of England following the death of King Stephen, who had presumed Henry to be his heir. Eleanor's marriage to Henry did not lack discord, and the couple argued often. However, they produced eight children before Eleanor separated from Henry in 1167 and moved her household to her lands in Poitiers. It is believed that Eleanor, being such a strong and energetic woman, would not stand for her husband's infidelities.

While Eleanor was mistress of her own lands, she encouraged a culture of chivalry among her courtiers that would long influence poetry, music, literature, and folklore. Eleanor's court attracted artists and poets, and it flourished for several years.

In 1173, Henry, one of Eleanor's sons, began plotting to seize the English throne from his father as he grew hungry for power. Eleanor, who was rumoured to be supporting her son, was arrested for treason and imprisoned. She spent the next sixteen years being moved around to different castles and strongholds in England and possibly playing a role in the death of her estranged husband's mistress. Young Henry, with seemingly little interest in government, spent the next decade charming the court with his personality and participating heavily in the tournament culture of the times.

Young Henry became ill with dysentery in 1183, and prior to his death that summer he begged his father to release Eleanor. The king agreed and allowed her to return to his household for part of the year. She was able to resume some of her duties as queen. When the king died in July of 1189, their son Richard (1157–1199) succeeded him. Richard completed the act of freeing his mother from prison, and she got her complete independence. Eleanor ruled as regent in her son's name while he went to lead the Third Crusade.

Richard (known as Richard the Lionheart) returned to rule England until his death in 1199. Eleanor's youngest son, John (1166–1216), was crowned king after the death of his brother, whom she would support against the rebellion of her grandson Arthur (1187–1203).

Eleanor of Aquitaine died in 1204, but she is still considered one of the most important women in English history. Her contributions to her nation extended well beyond her lifetime. She was tenacious, wise, and politically savvy, with a maturity that went well beyond her years. The nuns who were with her during her death at Fontevrault Monastery said: 'She was beautiful and just, imposing and modest, humble and elegant … a Queen who surpassed almost all the queens of the world.'

Henry Tudor and the Birth of a Dynasty

For those reigning, establishing legitimacy for the inheritance of the crown was absolutely crucial. A prime example of this is the reign of Henry VII of England (1457–1509).

Henry Tudor was born at Pembroke Castle in Wales to Lady Margaret Beaufort (1443–1509), who was only 13 years old at the time. Henry's father, Edmund Tudor (1430–1456), died three months before his birth. His mother, the heiress of the House of Beaufort, was the great-granddaughter of John of Gaunt, 1st Duke of Lancaster (1340–1399), which bolstered Henry's claim to the English throne. The House of Lancaster and the House of York both started with John of Gaunt and Edmund Langley (1341–1402), sons of Edward III (1312–1377).

The children of the House of Beaufort were legitimised as a sub-branch of the House of Lancaster by King Richard II (1367–1400) after the marriage of John of Gaunt to Katherine Swynford (1343–1409). This now meant that John Beaufort (1404–1444), Henry's maternal grandfather, had joined the line of succession after any legitimate children of John of Gaunt. Henry's mother became head of the House of Beaufort when neither her uncles nor brothers produced a male heir, leaving Henry Tudor as the rightful Lancastrian heir to the throne.

Some 400 years earlier, William the Conqueror (1028–1087) had established the right of conquest of the throne. In 1485, at the age of 28, Henry Tudor so defended his claim to the English throne by defeating the Yorkist King Richard III (1452–1485), in the Battle of Bosworth (1485). However, the Yorkists and the Lancastrians had been embroiled in the Wars of the Roses for over thirty years (1455–1485), so Henry needed to legitimise his right to kingship. In 1486, he married Elizabeth of York (1466–1503), niece of Richard III, thereby ending the Wars of the Roses and giving all their future children a place in the Yorkist and Lancastrian lines. Henry ensured he was the rightful ruler in every way, including Pope Innocent VIII (1432–1492) officially recognising his marriage to Elizabeth. Henry Tudor became Henry VII, and his children and grandchildren would do everything in their power to ensure his claim to the throne was not in vain.

Once Henry VII established the legitimacy of the crown, his entire future depended on the birth of a son and heir. Thankfully, his marriage to Elizabeth of York was fruitful, and the Tudor dynasty would continue for the next 118 years.

Throughout European history, the right of succession was almost always left to the eldest son or the nearest male relative. In the case of Henry VIII (1491–1547), son of Henry VII, it was his duty to see that a son carried on the Tudor dynasty. Despite marrying six times, he only had one surviving son and two surviving daughters. Henry drafted out the line of succession to ensure that should his son Edward (1537–1553) die or have no children, his eldest daughter Mary (1553–1558) would rule, and if she in turn had no children, then her half-sister Elizabeth (1558–1603) would follow. While Henry's dying wish was to see his dynasty continued by generations of male heirs, this was not the case.

Edward VI, the boy king, ascended to the throne in January of 1547, at the age of 9. He reigned until he was 15, as he died of consumption in July 1553. However, like his father, Edward was a Protestant reformer determined to keep Catholicism out of England. When Edward was on his deathbed, he changed his father's act of succession with the stroke of a pen. According to Henry's wishes, because Edward had no heirs his sister Mary was due to take the throne. But Mary was a devout Catholic who would undoubtedly bring her country back to what she believed was the true church if she reigned as queen. With the pressure of his regents, who were also in favour of a Protestant England, Edward changed the succession so his cousin Jane, would inherit the throne. Lady Jane Grey (1536–1554), also a Protestant, was queen for nine days following the death of Edward, but Mary Tudor and her powerful army took back the crown and Lady Jane was executed at the age of 16. For a short time, England did indeed return to Catholicism.

The Abolishment of the English Absolute Monarchy

The Golden Age of European monarchies would continue until 1750, but it didn't always run that smoothly. In 1629, things started to go south for Charles I of England (1600–1649) when he became caught up in a conflict with Parliament. Aside from conflicting ideas about religion, there was much displeasure over the king's economic policies and his use of power. Charles was an advocate for absolute monarchy and believed he should govern without the advice and consent of Parliament and promptly dissolved it. Parliament, however, insisted it played a necessary role in government.

When Charles came to the throne in 1625, he continued with custom duties granted to the crown since medieval times, such as tonnage and poundage for example, even though Parliament was against it. Tonnage and poundage began during the reign of Edward II and were a series of taxes on imported goods from Portugal and Spain. The rest of Charles' reign would not be a good one for in 1629, after dismissing parliament completely, he was forced to raise taxes again. Unrest in Scotland in 1641 caused the king to call on parliament to obtain funds for war with the Scots. The king's subjects in both England and Scotland protested the raising of taxes. By March of 1642, the Royalists, who sided with the king, and the Parliamentarians, supported by the Scots, formally declared war.

In 1646, after the Royalists were defeated, the king surrendered to the Scots as he feared being captured by the Parliamentary army. Despite pressure to sign the National Covenant, an agreement opposing the reforms of The Church of Scotland, King Charles refused and was then handed over to parliament. General Oliver Cromwell, a senior commander in the Parliamentary army, along with a group of parliament members felt there would be no peace in England as long as Charles was king.

In 1649, Charles was put on trial for being a traitor and a tyrant. The Parliamentarian High Court of Justice declared the king guilty of trying to 'uphold himself an unlimited and tyrannical power to rule according to his will and to overthrow the rights and liberties of the people'. He was sentenced to death by beheading and is the only English king to have been tried and executed for treason.

The monarchy was abolished after the execution of Charles I as Parliament felt that a king in England was unnecessary and dangerous to liberty and the public interest of the people. But the Scots were loyal to his son, Charles II (1630–1685) and declared him king. In 1650, Cromwell and his army defeated the Scots at The Battle of Dunbar and Charles II was then hunted throughout England for several months. In 1651, he fled for France under political asylum.

After being in exile at the Hague for almost ten years, Charles returned to England in 1660, and reclaimed the monarchy in what was known as the Restoration (1660–1688). The judges who signed the death warrant of Charles I were tried with regicide and executed. The British monarchy was back, but its powers were lessened, and in 1688, the constitutional monarchy in England was established.

The Sun King

Louis XIV of France (1638–1715) is a fine example of the grandeur of the absolute monarchy. As king, he understood the finer details of being a monarch, and the foundation of his kingdom made a great distinction between ceremonial greatness and actual power. His reign was so successful that he was referred to as The Sun King.

As king, Louis gave his ministers only symbolic authority, and even that depended on his every word. Instead of giving them actual power over matters, they were instead showered with decorative honours. This gave the illusion of worth, keeping the nobility busy while Louis had all the power as he kept the well-educated elites at his mercy. Perhaps Louis XIV was lucky in that he ruled during a time that was not as dangerous as it would be for his descendants. During eighteenth-century France, the ideas of the monarchy were challenged. Due to the lavish spending of both Louis XIV and his son, Louis XV (1710–1774), the French Monarchy fell under duress. In addition to the fortunes spent at Versailles, Louis XV gave considerable amounts of money to the American colonists, leaving his son with an unstable France.

In 1789, King Louis XVI (1754–1793) called the Estates General, a ruling body that represented all the people in France, in the hopes of raising money. The First Estate consisted of clergy, and the Second, nobles. The Third Estate was the other 95 per cent of France's population, mainly the workers and the oppressed. The First and Second Estates expected the king to grant them more power. However, he instead, expected them to hand over more taxes. They also refused to allow members of the Third Estate to attend the meetings, and so the Third Estate declared itself a National Assembly.

They met on the 20 June 1789 to draw up plans for a constitutional government. The Declaration of Rights of Man and the Citizens was drafted and adopted in August. The National Assembly was now part of France's new constitution and defined liberties to be had by all men. It also cancelled out the monarch's divine right, which had been in place since the ninth century.

The Three Estates had very different ideas on how to run things in France, and the king could not be bothered to sort them out. His total disregard for his people set the French Revolution in motion, and both Louis XVI and his Queen, Marie Antionette (1755–1793), were beheaded in 1793 for treason, ending the French Monarchy.

Not all monarchs were successful as Louis XIV or Henry Tudor. Nor did all monarchs have such a lengthy reign. After the Napoleonic Wars, the monarchy of France was briefly restored in 1814. However, Charles X of France (1757–1836) abdicated after his overthrow during the Revolution of 1830, leaving the throne to his son Louis. As he had no desire to be king, Louis-Antione XIX of France (1775–1844) would become the shortest reigning monarch – within twenty minutes of ascending the throne, he signed the necessary documents that he too may abdicate.

* * * *

Germany saw its last monarchy with Kaiser Wilhelm II (1859–1941), a great symbol of imperialist powers. In 1890, he wanted to dismiss Chancellor Otto von Bismark (1815–1898), who had united the German people and created the modern German states in 1862. The Kaiser also showed aggression towards Russia and France, and his desire for more political power ultimately led to Germany's involvement in World War One. In 1918, after Germany signed an armistice agreement, Kaiser Wilhelm II abdicated, ending the monarchy in Germany.

During this time, the end of another monarchy was approaching. In 1917, Tsar Nicholas II (1868–1918) was the absolute monarch of Russia, but he was weak and ineffective. During a 1905 uprising, he refused to listen to his people and create reforms that would have lessened the burdens of the poor.

During war with Germany, the Bolsheviks, a group of reformers led by Vladimir Lenin (1870–1924), seized control of Russia. They believed a violent overthrow of the monarchy was the answer to the country's problems.

Nicholas II was forced to abdicate, but the Bolsheviks still captured the Royal Family and confined them to a house in the city of Ekaterinburg. The Tsar was an important symbol in Russia and a threat to the Bolsheviks, as many Russians still supported the monarchy. In July 1918, Nicholas II and his family were brutally murdered. This caused not only the end of the monarchy, but also a Civil War.

Not all monarchs were successful as Louis XIV or Henry Tudor. Nor did all monarchs have such a lengthy reign. After the Napoleonic Wars, the monarchy of France was briefly restored in 1814. However, Charles X of France (1757–1836) abdicated after his overthrow during the Revolution of 1830, leaving the throne to his son Louis. King Louis-Antione XIX of France (1775–1844) would become the shortest reigning monarch as he had no desire to be king, and within twenty minutes, signed the documents needed that he too may abdicate the throne of France.

Although Finland never really had a royal family, it did technically have a king – if only for two months. Charles, the first King of Finland, became the country's first and last monarch in 1918. The country was under Swedish rule and then Russian rule from 1809–1917. Finland declared its independence from Russia in late 1917 but this only led to a bloody civil war. Pro-Finnish Whites, led by Baron Mannerheim, decided that the country could benefit from a king. German noble, Prince Fredrick Charles of Hesse, was elected in October 1918. While the Finnish people were not happy about a German King, Charles took his duty seriously. But when Kaiser Wilhelm abdicated in November of 1918, King Charles of Finland did the same due to political pressure. He never even set foot in his own kingdom.

Denmark has the longest reigning dynasty to date – more than 1,200 years, and it is still in place today. The Danish monarchy was founded in the eighth century with Gorm the Old (958), who ruled Denmark from 926 to 958 until his death. The current queen of Denmark, Margrethe II (1940–), can trace her lineage back to the first monarch.

Through the line of succession, the throne was issued for the sole purpose of keeping the family's bloodline strong throughout the dynasty. In most cases, especially in Europe, the heir was known ahead of time, and a smooth transition was hoped for. The eldest child of the king, usually a son, would be the first in line to the throne. If something were to complicate this, such as a death, the second son in line would rule. This was known as having 'an heir and a spare' and most families strived to have at least two healthy sons under their belt. Some European countries had a total exclusion of a female being able to rule, but this was not the case throughout the world.

Most future monarchs were brought up in a royal family where they were trained for their expected future reign. While royal parents were invested in their children's health and education, the daily care of the child was usually entrusted to others. Eleanor of Aquitaine's younger children were educated at Fontevraud Abbey in France, though she was not very involved in their day to day lives.

When Edward II (1284–1327) was born in 1284, it was believed he would be the next great king to bring England to victory over the Welsh. Edward was predeceased by three brothers, leaving him heir to the throne. He was given an official household with staff, which was common for reigning families. Edward was most likely educated by Dominican friars who became part of his household in 1290. He was also assigned a magister, who would oversee his discipline, as well as his training in military skills. Like several children in line for the throne, Edward was not allowed to take part in jousting for his personal safety.

Royal children were almost never raised at court with their parents, especially during the Middle Ages. Royal sons and daughters were both sent away to be educated by tutors and raised by a governess.

In some cases, a king would have his eldest son crowned during his lifetime, almost as a junior king. This was done in the case of Henry the Young, king of England (1155–1183), and in the House of Capet in France during 987–1328.

In some cases, joint sovereigns ruled together, as in the case of William III (1650–1702) and his wife, Mary II of England (1662–1694). Peter I (1672–1725) and his half-brother Ivan V (1666–1696) reigned Russia together in the late seventeenth and early eighteenth centuries. In 1516, Charles V (1500–1558) ruled Spain alongside his mother, Juana of Castile (1479–1555).

Many times, throughout European and world history, the throne was inherited by an heir at a very young age. Mary queen of Scots (1542–1587), became queen of Scotland at just six days old, after her father died of cholera. Scottish nobleman James Hamilton, 2nd Earl of Arran (1516–1575), was appointed regent on her behalf.

Alfonso XIII (1886–1941) was arguably the king of Spain while still in his mother's womb. His father, Alfonso XII (1857–1885), died in November of 1885, seven months before his birth. His mother, Maria Christina of Austria (1858–1929), served as regent until Alfonso was 16.

In the absence of an heir, the next most senior member of the family would assume the role of monarch. However, this caused problems upon the death of Edward IV (1422–1483). Edward fell ill in 1483 and died at the age of 40, perhaps from a stroke. His eldest son, Edward (1470–1483), who was 12 years old, was heir to the throne. Upon his deathbed, Edward IV instructed that his brother, Richard Duke of Gloucester, reign as regent until the boy was of age to rule. However, the young prince and his brother were soon imprisoned in the Tower of London and never seen again. The Duke of Gloucester claimed the throne for himself and has been wildly accused of being responsible for the death of his nephews.

George V (1865–1936), the grandfather of the late Queen Elizabeth II (1926-2022), passed away after a long illness in January 1936. His son Edward (1894–1972) became king of England upon the death of his father. However, Edward VIII would have a short and tumultuous reign. Just one month into his rule, he proposed marriage to American socialite Wallis Simpson (1896–1986), with whom he was deeply in love. Because Wallis was a divorced woman, several members of parliament greatly opposed the marriage. They argued that a divorced woman serving as queen consort would be unacceptable. It also went against the tenets of the Church of England. When it became clear to Edward that he could not remain on the throne and marry Mrs Simpson, he chose love. He abdicated in December 1936. Because Edward had no children, the throne of England was passed to his younger brother, George (1895–1952). The abdication caused turmoil in the royal family until Edward's passing in 1972.

Because the future of the monarchy was entirely dependent on the birth of a child, royal couples faced a tremendous amount of pressure from all sides to withhold the stability of their kingdom. The pressure to deliver a son and heir to a royal family fell almost wholly on the queen. Her success and reputation were defined by whether a healthy baby boy was born. If a royal couple found themselves unable to have children, it was almost always blamed on the queen. She could be accused of having lewd behaviour or deliberately disobeying the king. Henry VIII blamed his first and second wives for not producing a male heir even though they both gave birth to thriving baby girls.

Having several healthy sons was a promise to the country that God was pleased, and all was well in the kingdom. The Plantagenets stand out as a dynasty that produced generations of male heirs. As discussed earlier, Henry II, the first Plantagenet king, and his wife, Eleanor of Aquitaine, had five sons, and his heir, King John, had two sons. Henry III had six sons, and his son, Edward I, also had six sons. The reign of Plantagenet kings would produce more than twenty sons over a span of 150 years.

It's no secret that the pressure to produce a male heir and carry on the dynasty was all consuming. Kings and queens throughout time have gone to extensive lengths to be sure they had a healthy son, including pilgrimages and lengthy prayers. Monarchs throughout Europe's history probably didn't sleep well until they had at least one son.

Medieval Europe was a tapestry of royal families, and the transmission of power was by blood alone, not by election.

A successful dynasty needed to defend itself against rivals, ensure a strong bloodline and control any rivalry in the dynasty itself.

Some kings in the eleventh and twelfth centuries had many sons with different partners. Toirdelbach Ua Conchobair, king of Connacht Ireland (1088–1156), had six partners who together gave him 22 sons.

Toirdelbach was born in 1088 and ascended to the throne in 1106 with the assistance of his uncle. Roughly thirty years later, Toidelbach advanced the High Kingship and designated his son Conchobar Ua Conchobair (1126–1144) heir to the throne. But several of Toidelbach's other sons did not agree with this decision. Two of them, Aedh (1136–1194) and Ruadhri (1136–1198), staged a rebellion against their father in 1136, which led to their capture and imprisonment in 1143. It was a year later that Conchobar would be murdered before he could become king.

Toirdelbhach then chose another son, Domhnall Mor mac Tairrelbach (1144–1176), to be heir to the throne. However, Ruadhri was attempting to gain his father's attention by capturing his cousin, who had rebelled against the king. When Domhnall was arrested, Ruadhri's position as heir was restored, and he succeeded his father as king.

By learning about Toirdelbhach's turbulent reign, it's easy to understand how the abundance of male heirs caused friction. The drive to become king and claim the throne often led to dire consequences. Turmoil was often caused in the family, and kings and their heirs were sometimes killed by their family members as much as they could have been killed by outside forces.

By the early Middle Ages, the majority of royal families accepted the concept of marriage as defined through the Catholic Church. The church dominated daily life by all accounts and exercised tremendous influence over everyone, from serfs and merchants to the ruling monarch.

Because of St Augustine's influence in the Middle Ages, the church delegated itself as the authority on marriage. St Augustine was a skilled theologian with increasing importance who lived during the fourth and fifth centuries. The Church looked favourably upon marriage as not only a blessed union but a sacrament and was declared as such in 1184. Adultery was severely frowned upon and taking more than one wife was forbidden, which put considerable pressure on a reigning queen to produce an heir.

In royal families, the choice of a bride for a king or prince was almost purely political. Marriages were arranged to secure an alliance with a neighbouring country, and negotiations often began when royal children were very young. In 1518, a peace treaty was signed by England and France, leading to the betrothal of Henry VIII's 2-year-old daughter to Francis, the infant dauphin of France (1518–1536). Marie Antoinette married the dauphin of France, future King Louis XVI, in May of 1770 when she was just 14 but their marriage had been arranged several years prior. In 1548, 5-year-old Mary Queen of Scots was betrothed to Francis II of France (1544–1560), who was a young child himself. A marriage contract was signed, which stated that France and Scotland would be united under Mary and Francis.

Behind the motivation to preserve the family dynasty came a profound desire to please God. Because kings and queens of Europe felt they were chosen by God to rule, they also felt it was their duty to protect their bloodlines for years to come, which was even more reason to keep marriage prospects to a limited few.

The term 'blueblood', which ties in to preserving nobility in the royal family, originated from fifteenth-century Spain. From as early as the eighth century to the fifteenth century, the Moors – who were of Arabic descent – ruled over much of Spain; many interracial marriages occurred before their civilization crumbled and they were finally defeated. The last Muslim king, Boabdil the Unlucky (1460–1533), surrendered to King Ferdinand of Aragon (1452–1516) and Isabella I of Castile (1451–1504), the Catholic powerhouse that ruled over Spain in 1492. Both the king and queen of Spain were intolerant of any minorities and wanted interracial marriages with Moors to end.

The Spanish aristocrats, especially those in Castile, were also of a fair complexion and began to distinguish themselves from all others by calling themselves 'sangre azul'. Because their skin was so fair, the veins in their arms looked blue, which they associated with purity and nobility. They also deliberately avoided the sun to keep their skin light. Anyone with darker skin was either Moorish or lower class, as those working in the fields would have had their skin browned by the sun.

This trend continued throughout Europe as nobles were often defined by their pale skin and blue veins. Royals went to great lengths to preserve the blue bloods throughout their dynasty, yet another reason why royal intermarriage was so prevalent.

However, close royal intermarriage and inbreeding didn't just occur in Europe. George III, one of the world's most recognisable kings, was the product of inbreeding, and one of the most powerful dynasties in history was overflowing with genetic mutations that spanned centuries.

Chapter Three

Ancient Egypt, The Roman Empire, and The Ptolemy Dynasty

The history of Ancient Egypt extends beyond the reach of written record. After King Narmer united Egypt's upper and lower kingdoms, the Egyptian people made great advancements, including the development of Hieroglyphics and the solar calendar. The people of the Nile consolidated political power and economic development. Improved agricultural strategies were followed by advances in irrigation and drainage. Between 2630 and 2528 bce, the first pyramid was designed by the architect Imhotep, followed by others, including the Great Pyramid of Giza. The dominant city of Heliopolis gained stature, and its god, Re, was introduced into the pantheon.

With the upper and lower kingdoms united, King Narmer also established a central government in Ancient Egypt. Egyptian society thrived on the construction of religion and government working as a whole. The structure of temples and the creation of taxes, laws, labour, trade, and defences were managed by social hierarchy. Pharaohs maintained religious harmony throughout the kingdom and oversaw all that went on.

Like so many of the European royal families that would come after them, the Ancient Egyptians practised inbreeding to keep their bloodlines pure. It was a very common practice, and royals were expected to marry within the family. Women were believed to carry the royal blood of the family, and it was customary for the eldest son and daughter of the pharaohs to marry, often becoming co-rulers. Pharaohs their nieces; it is believed that they practised this 'double niece method' because their god Osiris was married to his sister, Isis, to keep the bloodline pure.

Tutankhamun (1341–1323 BC) ruled during the New Period of Ancient Egyptian History and is thought to come from a long line of inbreeding. Tutankhamen was born around 1341 BC during the late Eighteenth Dynasty. Though his actual year of birth is debatable, he probably lived within the time frame of 1360–1340 BC. He was born during the reign of Akhenaten (1363–1361 BC), who was believed to be his father. Akhenaten most likely co-ruled with his wife, Nefertiti (1370–1330 BC), or his daughter Meritaten. There is still some dispute as to who Tutankhamen's mother was. Some have suggested that his mother was a woman named Meketaten, the second daughter of King Akhenaten and Nefertiti. But this seems unlikely as Meketaten was around 10 years old when she died. Some have concluded that Nefertiti was not Tutankhamun's mother and that his mother may have been his sister Meritaten.

A genetic examination carried out in 2008 on Tutankhamun's remains and the remains of others do indicate that his father was Akhenaten. The analysis also determined that his mother was his father's full sister. Other researchers believe that Nefertiti was his mother but that she was a cousin of Akhenaten. While it remains impossible to tell for sure, the DNA samples taken of Tutankhamun's parents concluded that there was indeed a genetic closeness and that they were either brother and sister, or first cousins.

DNA tests also concluded that Tutankhamun's grandparents were Pharaoh Amenhotep III (1401–1353 BC) and his wife, Tiye (1398–1338 BC). Tutankhamun's father was the heir to the throne when Amenhotep passed. The same DNA tests state that Tutankhamun's mother was one of the five daughters born to Amenhotep and Tiye, making her Akhenaten's sister. Tutankhamun's family's incestuous trend would continue into his reign.

Tutankhamun probably came into power around 1332 BC, and that same year, he married his half-sister Ankhesenamun (1348–1322 BC), daughter to his father Akhenaten, and his queen, Nefertiti.

While not much is known about his personal life, Tutankhamun was most likely raised in his father's court, and we know that his early years are centred around the city of Thebes, a civilization that throbbed with life. As a boy, Tutankhamun attended school as most Egyptian children were taught to read by the age of 4. He would have been taught to recognise hieroglyphics, use figures, and do mental arithmetic. Because it would have been affordable to the young prince's family, he would have used papyruses to write on.

Tutankhamun became king when he was 9 years old and was escorted to his coronation by the highest of court dignitaries. The elaborate ceremony made him king of all people, and as he sat on an ancient throne, the crowns of the North and the South were placed on his small head.

Because he was so young when beginning his reign, he would serve alongside chief advisors. Ay, an elderly official who had long been with Tutankhamun's family, was one of his top advisors. Throughout his reign, Tutankhamun restored temples along with the privileges of the old gods. He also repaired several sacred shrines which had been damaged during the reign of his father.

Tutankhamun and his wife had only two daughters, both stillborn. Inbreeding often resulted in stillbirths, genetic disorders, and defects. The inbreeding between his parents had certainly taken a toll on the king. Depictions of Tutankhamun show him with an oddly shaped head and a womanly body, including developed breasts. His face regularly shows that he had swollen lips and a very thin nose.

But if one looks closely at the mask of Tutankhamun, it can be very deceiving. The smooth, perfectly symmetrical face and large almond-shaped eyes are set between high cheekbones. Though his lips are full, they are not swollen. They are more sensuous, almost childlike. His face looks serene and confident, with the slightest hint of a smile. These elegant and delicate features make Tutankhamun appear flawless and beautiful.

But these depictions were far from the truth. The boy king suffered greatly because of his family's inbreeding, enduring a host of afflictions throughout his reign.

Through years of research, scientists are almost certain that Tutankhamun, who is estimated to have stood around 5½ ft tall, had a form of scoliosis – a curvature of the spine usually diagnosed today during adolescence through exams and X-ray. It is still not clear today why children develop this disorder, and most cases are fairly mild. Those diagnosed are closely monitored, and surgery may be necessary in serious cases. However, some cases of scoliosis can greatly hinder day-to-day life; the severity of the spinal curve often changes the amount of space in the chest necessary for the lungs to function, leading to breathing problems. In the case of Tutankhamun, it's quite possible his scoliosis was debilitating, especially since there would have been little understanding of the disorder or treatment at the time.

While studying his remains, a U-shaped headrest was discovered. Scientists think it may have been a pillow made for the king to help support his head and spine, perhaps coaxing his spine to lay straighter. One of the stillborn daughters buried with her father shows evidence of being afflicted with the same condition.

Researchers took several CT scans of Tutankhamun's remains and discovered that he also had severe kyphoscoliosis – a curvature of both the coronal and sagittal plates of the spine. He was also found to have a deformity of the toe, which is believed to have been caused by the curvature of the spine. Scientists assume that Tutankhamun must have been in considerable pain when walking. Most drawings of the king depict him in a chariot, which was unusual at the time. An estimated 130 walking sticks were found in the king's tomb. It was originally believed that the sticks depicted his power or royalty, but most Egyptologists today believe they may have been a form of a crutch or a cane. Because his spine was uneven, it's possible that he had difficulty walking or standing without the assistance of one of his canes. Some paintings found in his tomb show him leaning on his cane with his leg tucked behind him. Another possible reason for the walking sticks is that he was thought to have been afflicted by a club foot, another trait which may have been due to genetics or inbreeding.

Researchers who studied the DNA of Tutankhamun and his family found an abundance of malformations. Pathologies suggesting Kohler Disease, a bone disorder of the foot usually seen in children. While the disease is rare, it greatly affects males over females. The condition causes painful swelling along the length of the foot arch and usually does not affect both feet. The flow of blood to the navicular bone in the foot gets interrupted, leading to a degeneration of the bone. Putting weight on the affected foot causes pain, and walking is difficult if the condition is not treated. As with scoliosis, Tutankhamun would not have had proper treatment of any foot ailment, whether it was Kohler Disease or a clubbed foot.

Like his father, Tutankhamun also suffered from a partial cleft palate. While it appeared that he was well fed and well cared for as a king most certainly would have been, his crooked teeth were characteristic of those who shared his bloodline. His relatively large front incisors and overbite were both seen in his elders. Research also states that the king suffered from an impacted wisdom tooth, although there did not appear to be an infection. If he had suffered from a tooth infection, it would likely have contributed to his death.

While Tutankhamun's health problems resulted from years of inbreeding, they were not the immediate cause of his death. Some research suggests that his death was partially caused by a gangrenous infection in his leg, which may have been the result of a severe break. DNA tests along with tomography show that he suffered from a terrible case of malaria as well, which may have also contributed to his death.

When we envision Tutankhamun today, we associate him with his death mask and a face that is hauntingly beautiful. The glowing gold representing the skin of the divine, and the command of those black eyes framed with ornamented blue eyebrows gives the image of a muscular and youthful king. When looking at his death mask, there are no suggestions that he lived a life filled with disease and physical ailments. But like most kings, Tutankhamun is an image conjured up by artists of the time whose job was to present the powerful, almighty ruler who was the epitome of perfection during his time.

Inbreeding was still practised throughout Ancient Egypt for several centuries after the death of Tutankhamun. Perhaps the most notorious being the Ptolemy dynasty – the family of Cleopatra VII. The Ptolemaic dynasty ruled the Ptolemaic kingdom during the Hellenistic period, from 305 to 30 BC, and was the last family to rule Ancient Egypt.

The Ptolemies were believed to be successors to the Macedonian king, Alexander the Great (356–323 BC). While in battle, Ptolemy I (367–282 BC) was Alexander's general, and according to some, his half-brother. When Alexander died and his empire was divided, Egypt fell into the lap of Ptolemy, who became the first ruler of the Ptolemaic dynasty. The dynasty was quick to fall into the same vicious circle of intermarriage, which had likely given Tutankhamun many of his afflictions many centuries before.

But the first full-scale marriage of siblings of this dynasty is seen with Ptolemy's son, Ptolemy II (309-246 BC), who married his sister, Arsinoe II (316-270 BC), although they did not produce an heir. Arsinoe was initially married to the king of Thrace (360-281 BC) when she was a teenager. However, her life was often in danger, and she made several attempts at escaping. She knew she could not trust anyone outside the family if she wanted to be safe. She left her husband, returned to Egypt, and married her brother Ptolemy. By marrying her brother, she was able to secure the link between the new Ptolemaic dynasty and the traditions of her native Egypt. Her thought process would certainly serve her well, as she would become the first female Pharaoh of the dynasty. Arsinoe II would rule not just as the king's wife but in her own right as well. Perhaps it was here that the tradition of incest took hold. Maybe it was understood that it served a political purpose to strengthen what was essentially a new dynasty.

Ptolemy III (280–222 BC) – Ptolemy II's son from his previous marriage to Arsinoe I (305-248) – married his half-cousin, Berenice II (266–221 BC), the daughter of Magas of Cyrene (317-250 BC) and the reigning queen of Cyrenaica, Apama II (292-249 BC,) thereby welcoming her territory into the Ptolemaic dynasty.

The Ptolemy family had begun a long tradition of intermarriage that carried through the generations. Two of the children of Ptolemy III, Ptolemy IV (244-204 BC) and his sister Arsinoe III (245-204), would marry and have a son, Ptolemy V (210–180 BC), who would be the first child of a full-sibling marriage in the Ptolemy dynasty.

Ptolemy IV was around twenty years old when he was crowned. His mother was said to have supported his younger brother, Magas (241-221), instead of Ptolemy IV himself. Magas was popular with the army as he held significant military commands. Perhaps it was because of this favouritism that Magas would be scalded to death in his bathtub and that Berenike II would die shortly afterwards, supposedly by poison.

The son of Ptolemy IV, Ptolemy V, inherited the throne at only 5 years old when both of his parents died. Ptolemy's reign would fall under collapse, as well as initiate the transfer of power under the Roman conquest.

Ptolemy V married his third cousin, Cleopatra I (204–176 BC), and they produced two sons and one daughter. Their oldest son, Ptolemy VI (186–145 BC), married his sister, Cleopatra II (185–116 BC), and their union produced several children. After falling from his horse in battle, Ptolemy VI died at a young age from a fractured skull. His widowed wife, Cleopatra II, then married her other brother, Ptolemy VIII (184–116 BC) during a revolution in Alexandria.

The reign of Ptolemy VIII has been viewed as a complete disaster. Ptolemy himself was known as a tyrannical beast with the nickname 'Physcon', meaning fatty or potbelly, as his indulgence in luxurious foods caused him to become morbidly obese. Ptolemy VIII entered into his new marriage by immediately killing his nephew (and son of his new wife) Ptolemy VII. Whether or not Ptolemy VII actually reigned is controversial and historians believe it was unlikely that he was ever king, though he was given royal dignity after his death. Ptolemy VIII most likely saw his nephew as a rival to the throne and a threat to his rule. Still covered in the blood of his nephew, Ptolemy VIII came to the marriage bed to consummate the union. Understandably, Cleopatra II loathed her new husband and brother, but despite this, she soon gave birth to their first child, Memphites.

In keeping with his vile nature, Ptolemy VIII then raped one of his wife's daughters (the sister to the nephew he had murdered), and when she became pregnant, he took her as a second wife, and she also became a queen, Cleopatra III (160–101 BC).

Cleopatra II and her daughter, Cleopatra III, would rule alongside Ptolemy VIII until he died. Their triple reign was far from perfect, and at one point, Cleopatra II ousted both her daughter and husband from Alexandria before ruling alone for a time. In vengeance for doing so, Ptolemy VIII murdered their son, Memphites, who was only 12 years old. Ptolemy VIII dismembered his son's body and put it in a box before giving it to his wife on her birthday.

Ptolemy VIII had proved that he was maniacal. While some say he murdered his son as a form of ire against his wife, it is more than likely that he feared Memphites as yet another threat to the throne. Ptolemy VIII was obsessed with power and more than likely feared that his wife would attempt to co-rule with their son after banishing him from Alexandria. Ptolemy VIII went on to father two other sons with his second wife, Cleopatra III.

Cleopatra III would inherit the throne of Egypt after the death of Ptolemy VIII and her mother, which soon followed. She would find herself with a choice between her two sons, as both wanted to co-rule the empire with her. Each son felt it should be they who ruled alongside their mother, but it has been said that Cleopatra III felt nothing but hatred for her older son, Ptolemy IX (143–81 BC). She was insistent that he divorce his wife, Cleopatra IV (138–112 BC), who was also his sister, with whom he was very in love, and marry his other sister Cleopatra Selene (135–69 BC). Cleopatra III much preferred her younger son, Ptolemy X Alexander (140–88BC); he, however, ended up committing matricide as he was tired of his mother's demanding ways.

Ptolemy X Alexander then married his niece Cleopatra Berenike III (120-80 BC), the daughter of his brother Ptolemy IX Lathyros and their sister Cleopatra IV. When Ptolemy X Alexander died, Lathyros came to the throne with his daughter, Cleopatra Berenike III. When Lathyros died, Cleopatra Berenike III would go on to rule with her cousin and stepson, Ptolemy XI (105-80 BC). There is some speculation that she was actually his mother and not his stepmother, though we cannot be certain.

The throne of Ancient Egypt was then passed to Ptolemy XII Auletes (117–51 BC), son of Ptolemy XI. Historians aren't sure who Auletes's mother was, though it is possible he was the child of his father's beloved sister/wife, Cleopatra IV.

Ptolemy XII Auletes married Cleopatra V Tryphaina (57 BC), who was believed to have been his sister – though we can't be sure whether it was a full sister or a half-sister.

This prolonged string of inbreeding leads us to the most famous of the Egyptian queens, Cleopatra VII (69–30 BC). We know that XII Auletes (117–51 BC) was her father, but the subject of who her mother was, is debatable. Her mother may have been Cleopatra V, or possibly one of her father's other wives or even a concubine. However, going by her birthday, it seems the most logical person would be Cleopatra V.

We know Cleopatra VII married both of her brothers, though we can't sure whether it was in succession. Her younger brother Ptolemy XIII (62–47 BC) was killed during the Alexandrian War, and it's believed that Cleopatra murdered her younger brother, Ptolemy XIV (59–44 BC), because she wanted a path to the throne for her own son, who was conceived with her lover, Julius Caesar (100–44 BC). It is not believed that any of Cleopatra's children were the product of incest and that the marriages with her brothers most likely weren't consummated.

Cleopatra VII has fascinated us for centuries, first through the plays of Shakespeare, then television and movies. Cleopatra VII was born in 69 BC and would be the first in her family to speak Egyptian.

She is renowned for her mysterious Eastern beauty, and it was said she could seduce any lover with her beautiful face and seductive eyes.

But historians think Cleopatra's looks may have reflected her family's lineage of inbreeding more than we realise. After creating a model of the queen based on coins and statues of her family members, archaeologist, Diana Preston presents the Egyptian beauty quite differently than today's cinema has done. Could Cleopatra possibly have the same traits as her family, such as a plump face and body (the family was known for obesity), a hawkish nose, and protruding chin? Many now say it was not her beauty that won people over, but her wit and intelligence.

When she was born, the Egyptian kingdom was under a great deal of pressure from the Romans as they struggled to keep their power. After a time in exile, Cleopatra's father was put back on the throne, taking his then 17-year-old daughter, Cleopatra VII, to rule alongside him. When her father died in 51 BC, Cleopatra was supposed to share the throne with her brother, and husband, Ptolemy XIII. Unfortunately for her, her brother disputed this arrangement; a great deal of fighting broke out between them and Cleopatra fled the palace.

After landing in Alexandria in pursuit of the Roman general Pompey, it would be Julius Caesar who would help Cleopatra win back her throne. After Pompey was found and executed by Cleopatra's brother, Caesar decided he would stay in Egypt, as Rome depended on the country for their grain. He felt that keeping the monarchy stable was in his favour.

While Ptolemy XIII was convinced he could make Julius Caesar see him as the sole ruler of Egypt, his sister had other plans. After sneaking back into the palace and essentially throwing herself at Julius's feet, Cleopatra was able to get Caesar on her side. While it seems to be up for debate among historians, the general story is that Cleopatra smuggled herself into the palace after being rolled up into a carpet. One of the palace assistants carried the rug over his shoulder, laid it before Caesar and unrolled the beautiful young queen before him.

The following morning when Ptolemy XIII woke up, he found out that his sister had somehow got into the palace and managed to persuade Caesar to support her as queen. Before a formal assembly, Caesar made it clear that he expected Cleopatra and her 13-year-old brother to rule together. He would soon become intimate with Cleopatra, and she would give birth to a son, Caesarion.

Ptolemy XIII died in 47 BC and was replaced as co-ruler by his younger brother, Ptolemy XIV. However, Cleopatra now had a son, which made her powerful. She would have Ptolemy XIV killed so her child could become her co-ruler. She saw herself as a powerful semi-divine mother to the new Egyptian king as she closely identified with the goddess Isis.

Julius Caesar was assassinated only a few years later in 44 BC, and in 41 BC, Mark Anthony (83-30 BC), now ruling the eastern part of the Roman Republic, beckoned Cleopatra to Asia Minor. She arrived in her royal barge with a massive golden stern, complete with lavender sails that billowed out behind her as she relaxed on a couch. As the pipes played and the incense burned, it is said that she was representative of Aphrodite. An awe-struck Anthony climbed aboard her vessel and returned to Egypt with her. He was smitten by the lavish gifts bestowed upon him as they dined. He questioned why she had not supported his troops while trying to fight Caesar's assassins. She assured Anthony that she had a fleet assembled, but they could not reach Caesar in time.

Anthony was captivated by Cleopatra's brilliance and her supposed beauty; this 40-year-old man was reduced to acting like a schoolboy. Anthony soon had only one priority: Cleopatra. The two fell in love and had three children together. They also aligned politically, and Cleopatra aided him with supplies when he was at war with the Parthians. After another disastrous war with Octavian (63 BC – AD 14), the ruler of the western part of the Roman Republic, Anthony and Cleopatra's fate was sealed as Octavian marched on Alexandria, the capital of Egypt.

The two would essentially die together. Anthony, believing Cleopatra had taken her own life, stabbed himself and was brought to her while still alive. But Cleopatra had not yet taken her own life, and when Anthony arrived, she laid him down on a soft bed. While referring to him as her husband and master, she tore at her flesh until she drew blood. Knowing that she would be taken into Rome by Octavian and showed off as a war trophy, she decided to take her own life.

After dressing herself in her most beautiful clothing, she climbed into a sarcophagus filled with sweet-smelling perfumes and lay next to Anthony, along with poisonous snakes, and together, they welcomed death.

For a woman who came from such a long line of inbreeding, how could Cleopatra have been as accomplished as she was? Compared to the disastrous reigns engulfed in intermarriage that came before and after her, she faired quite well.

She is remembered for being wickedly intelligent and perfectly crafted in using her alluring ways to get what she wanted. She was a powerful world conqueror who was always one step ahead of her opponents. While her impressive education may have given her a chance to learn several languages, it was her brilliance that allowed her to negotiate alliances and treaties with neighbouring nations. Cleopatra came from a Greek dynasty of pharaohs, but she was the only one to bother learning the Egyptian language. In reference to her ability to speak many languages, the Greek biographer Plutarch (AD 46–119) once commented on Cleopatra's voice, saying, 'she was like an instrument of many strings. She could pass from one language to another'. Because she spoke several languages, this allowed her more leverage when discussing alliances and treaties with other nations.

For centuries, incest dominated the marriage patterns of the Ptolemaic dynasty, so how could the heirs carry on such success? There is no doubt that centuries of these people were genetically compromised, which should have resulted in reduced fertility, genetic disorders, and an increase in infant or child mortality. The inbreeding should have rendered the family infertile after a period of time. And yet it didn't.

But is it just physical defects that stem from inbreeding? Or is the mind affected as well? As we dive deeper into the European royals who practised these close relations, we will see that both the body and the mind are affected. In Cleopatra's case, it's certainly possible that today she would have been diagnosed with serious mental instability. Her unstable and unhealthy relationships with men, especially Anthony, indicate a personality disorder. She had a history of impulsive, egotistic behaviour that often resulted in fits of rage if she didn't get her way. Her emotions shifted rapidly from fear to ecstasy to madness, and she had a history of suicidal threats, ultimately leading to her suicide.

Only a handful of generations after Cleopatra VII, we see Caligula (AD 12-41), a distant relative of Mark Anthony. Caligula is remembered for his questionable antics and possible incestual relationships with siblings. At just 24 years of age, Caligula became the sole emperor of Rome, and while his first six months as ruler were favourable, everything changed when he became ill. He was so ill that it was feared that he may die, but he did recover in October of AD 37 – though he was now almost unrecognisable.

Historians will debate that Caligula was intentionally poisoned or perhaps suffered from a mental breakdown, but in any event, he became a truly paranoid individual. His personality almost completely changed as everyone around him irritated him so much that he often killed those who displeased him, including his cousin. Landowners were reprimanded for no reason, and Caligula took their belongings; he had two of his men executed when they forgot his birthday. He was erratic and unpredictable and believed himself to be a living god. He was also known to thrown extravagant sex orgies which included his sisters and he is also believed to have raped several women.

Today, historians suggest that he may have suffered from epilepsy or hyperthyroidism, causing him debilitating headaches. It's also possible he suffered from bipolar disorder. However, whatever it was that ailed Caligula needs to be questioned for the possibility that it may have been a result of being from an inbred family, or simply one that just carried poor genetics.

Caligula was also the uncle of Nero (AD 37–68), as his younger sister, Agrippina (AD 15–59), was Nero's mother. Agrippina the Younger was born in AD 15, but when she just 4 years old, her father Germanicus Julius Caesar died suddenly and with some controversy – suggesting a possible bout of jealousy on the part of his uncle, Tiberius.

At 13 she married her older cousin, Gnaues Domitius Ahenobarbus (17 BC – AD 41). It is unknown if she was forced to take part in her brother's supposed sexual activities with his sisters, but we do know that she gave birth to her son, Lucius Domitius Ahenobarbus, known as Nero.

Nero, who would claim the Roman throne in AD 54, still carries with him the reputation of being a tyrannical and bloodthirsty man. He is responsible for killing his mother but there are contradictions for the motive. Some say that Nero killed his mother because of her plot to have him replaced with his second cousin.

At 24, he divorced his first wife and had her suffocated in a hot bath after having her wrists slit. She was then decapitated. He went on to murder his second wife and unborn child by kicking her in the stomach while pregnant. Nero also shared his uncle's bizarre sexual appetite.

We know Nero's parents were cousins, but it is also possible that Caligula was not only his uncle but also his father, given Caligula's lavish sexual escapades with his sisters. And is the behaviour of Caligula and Nero just a continuation of the atrocities in the Ptolemaic dynasty? Fairly strong evidence remains that the Romans still practised intermarriage, despite the rules against it. After the fall of the Western Roman Empire, the Ostrogothic Kingdom at Ravenna was established and Theodoric the Great prohibited intermarriage between the Romans.

Overall, sexual reproduction, especially in royalty, is a form of propaganda, and it is the enhancement of the species (in this case, the family) through evolution. Those with good genetics should be able to carry them on, and those with unfavourable genes would hopefully die off over time.

The danger of inbreeding, particularly with siblings, is that there are more chances for recessive genes to be manifested in the offspring as brothers and sisters carry much of the same genetic material. Recessive genes are noxious as they have been cleaned from the breeding population the way dominant genes have, but a dominant gene has more of a chance of killing off those who inherit the disease, preventing it from being passed on. Recessive genes don't really die out; they tend to lurk around. However, the consistent inbreeding in the Ptolemaic family meant they were more likely to produce genetic complications, but the combination of genetic material passed down is random, not certain. Today, studies of inbreeding worldwide are mostly of first-cousin marriages, as brother and sister marriages are not nearly as common. So, while disease, deformities and death are more likely in close inbreeding, it doesn't mean they would appear in every child.

The moral depravity of these ancient families was certainly evident. The effects of inbreeding caused the Ptolemies to be selfish, murderous, vengeful, and greedy. Was Cleopatra VII's erratic character due to the years of consistent inbreeding? Along with what was probably a form of mental illness, Cleopatra seemed to have no moral compass, so was murdering her siblings a family trait? Is it likely she inherited a set of chromosomes that almost 'programmed' her to murder her siblings? These traits could suggest that there is a mental imbalance in the family.

What about the physical defects of the family? Regarding reproduction and infant mortality rates, the Ptolemaic family didn't seem to have a huge problem. Ptolemy V was noted in history as very athletic and fit, and while he passed away at a young age, he had three healthy children. Cleopatra III, the product of brother-sister incest, who also married an uncle, had five children.

One member of the family who stuck out physically was Ptolemy VIII, who was said to have an enormous pot belly and an ugly face. He was short and unattractive, but was he the only one? Considering the time in ancient history we are dealing with, I'm keen to think it possible that Ptolemy VIII was one of the only members of the family to look 'out of the ordinary'. If the generations of the family had no obvious defects or abnormalities, there wouldn't have been anything for scribes to note.

Most royal incest was considered socially acceptable at the time, and although probably not overly desirable, there were enough such relationships to be able to produce an heir. Marriage within the family to continue royal lineage was seen as a form of duty.

In the Ptolemaic dynasty, another advantage of intermarriage was that it limited the influence of any foreign powers. Yet, as we saw, marriage to your siblings and cousins presents its own set of problems. Familiarity also breeds contempt, which was proven in the dynasty's urge to murder their own in favour of advancing political power.

If we move forward in time to the great dynasties of Europe, the notion of keeping the bloodline strong did not falter. While the instances of slaughtering your kin seemed to dwindle, the problems stemming from intermarriage and genetic abnormalities did not.

Chapter Four

The House of Valois and Lancaster and Two Mad Kings

The history of European monarchs is not without those who suffered debilitating mental illness. When the promise of relief was almost unheard of, one was often subject to humiliation and isolation. Nobles may have been able to afford a visit from a physician in the hopes that a good purge may rid them of their madness, but that still didn't change the fact that mental illness didn't discriminate and was easily passed through generations.

Today we understand much more about how the mind works and can take tremendous measures to treat the mentally ill. One thing that modern medicine has shown us is that mental illness is quite often hereditary. And when those genes are compromised in the form of inbreeding, the stakes are even higher.

If we look at the House of Valois, King Charles VI (1368–1422) stands out as the most mentally incompetent monarch. But if we look at his mother and father, perhaps we can understand where some of this mental instability came from.

The Valois dynasty was the royal house of France from 1328 to 1589, and they ruled the nation from the end of the feudal period through the early modern age. Charles V (1338–1380) was crowned king of France in 1364, and much of his reign would be dominated by the long and drawn-out Hundred Years' War with England (1337–1453).

Charles V would marry his cousin, Joanna of Bourbon (1338–1378), at just 12 years old. Though they were both young, the couple had a relatively strong marriage. But it was Joanna who may have carried the gene for mental illness that would plague her family for generations to come.

In December of 1368, Charles VI was born at the royal residence of the Hotel Saint-Pol in Paris as the Dauphin of France. Joanna was known as a mentally fragile woman who may have suffered from postpartum depression. After the birth of her son Louis (1372–1407) in 1372, her mental health suffered terribly. Charles was so concerned for his wife that he made a pilgrimage to pray for her recovery.

In 1378, Joanna died two days after the birth of her daughter, Catherine (1378–1388). Charles was devastated and made no attempt to hide his sorrow at her funeral. While showing grief was frowned upon at the time, Charles may have been an overly sensitive individual, and I think it's only fair to say that he was overtaken by sadness rather than suffering from any great depression. But if he was, his offspring may have had a greater chance of inheriting it as their parents were second cousins. I've found no compelling evidence to suggest that any of the couple's children, other than Charles VI, suffered from mental illness. Though Catherine died at the young age of 10, it may or may not have been a result of her parents' relationship as cousins, as the causes are unknown.

In 1380, leaving his son a favourable situation in the Hundred Years' War, Charles V died. Charles VI would sit on the throne at only 11 years of age, under the regency of his two uncles. The young king was said to be friendly and physically fit, as he enjoyed hunting and jousting.

By the age of 17, Charles had grown into a handsome man with gentle brown eyes and a strong nose. And he was ready to marry. While attending the wedding of a French Noble, Charles was seen making the rounds with guests and participating in a joust, as if to show off his charisma.

A marital match was suggested between the king and 14-year-old Isabeau of Bavaria (1370–1435). She was said to be intelligent and quick-witted and willingly absorbed her lessons on the etiquette of the French Court. As was customary for the time, she was to be examined nude before a marriage to the king would be approved. The strong-minded teenager stood motionless while being examined, which exhibited flawless behaviour for a future queen.

When the couple met in 1385, Charles was smitten with his beautiful new wife-to-be with her dark features, and they were married three days later. The king said: 'happiness and love entered his heart, for he saw that she was beautiful and young, and thus he greatly desired to gaze at her and possess her'.

She was given a lavish coronation ceremony, and people rejoiced over the new young couple. The king pampered his wife with gifts in their first year of marriage, including a red velvet saddle for her palfrey that was lined with copper and ornately decorated with the couple's initials. He gave her clothing, expensive tableware, and several rings. Charles was happy and in love, so it was natural for his physicians to be bewildered when the king suddenly fell ill in 1392.

Michel Pintouin, a St Denis monk (1350–1421), noted the events. The first reported illness took place in March of that year, and the king suffered: 'a chaude malaise from over-heated humours. He lost consciousness for a time and complained of severe chest pain that felt like a sword piercing through his heart.'[1]

The king seemed to recover within the month but would fall ill again in July that same year. A murder attempt on the life of his close friend and advisor, Olivier de Clisson (1336–1407), was made. Though he survived, the king was hell-bent on punishing the accused, Pierre de Craon (1345–1409). Because de Craon had taken asylum in Brittany, Charles prepared a military expedition when John V, Duke of Brittany (1389–1482), refused to hand him over.

At the beginning of the campaign on 1 July, Charles appeared to have a fever, and his speech was incoherent. His army's progress was slow, which caused him to exhibit clear impatience. Over a month later, the king and his men were travelling through the woods near Le Mans when a leper dressed in rags and bare feet suddenly appeared before them. He grabbed the bridle of the king's horse and shouted: 'Ride no further, noble King! Turn back as you are betrayed!'[2]

The king's men hit the leper but did not arrest or kill him. He continued to follow the king's procession through the forest for another half an hour. One of the king's pages, feeling overwhelmed by the heat of the hot August sun, suddenly dropped his lance, which then clanged loudly against the helmet of another page.

The king, reacting to the sound, drew his sword and yelled: 'Forward against the traitors! They wish to deliver me to the enemy.'[3]

The king spurred his horse and began to swing his sword frantically, killing several of his own men in the process. He continued to swing until a group of his soldiers and his chamberlain were able to subdue him. They pulled him from his horse and lay him on the ground. His men stood around and watched as the king simply lay still and had no reaction before falling into a coma. As a measure of caution, he was quickly brought to the castle of Creil in Northern France to recover, as it was thought that the fresh air and lovely surroundings might help.

Charles VI would lay in a coma for three days in Creil. His eyes continued to roll back in his head, and he recognised none of his men. His physicians were in fear for his life and tried to decipher whether the king had been poisoned, was suffering from overheated bile, or had been the victim of witchcraft. One of his venerated physicians, 92-year-old Guillaume de Harcigny (1300–1393), who had previously cared for his mother, recognised the symptoms, and concluded that the king had: 'inherited the moistness of the brain from his mother'.[4]

It would take a month before the king would return to full consciousness and recover. But he eventually regained awareness and was returned to Paris.

The following June, he suffered from another attack that lasted about six months and would set the stage for the next three decades of his condition. His illness was described as so severe that he was 'far out of the way; no medicine could help him'.[5]

The king would suffer from over forty episodes of mental illness throughout his life, which the monk of St Denis carefully recorded. The king's health deteriorated to the point where he did not recognise his own family. During an episode in 1393, he didn't know his name or that he was king of France. When his wife came to his chambers to visit, he no longer recognised her. He asked his servants who she was and then requested that she be led out of the room and leave him alone. While he demanded that the queen be kept away from him during his illness, he did allow her to act on his behalf, giving her much more power than was usually given to a medieval queen.

When the king first became ill, Isabeau was 22 years old with three children and the death of two infants on her heart. The monk of St Denis also described her pain at seeing the king in his state: 'What distressed her above all was to see how on all occasions ... the king repulsed her, whispering to his people, "Who is this woman obstructing my view? Find out what she wants and stop her from annoying and bothering me."'[6]

The king often complained of stabbing pain in his body and would then run through the palace at Hotel Saint-Pol until he collapsed from exhaustion. Servants would close off entrances to keep the king from escaping.

In 1395 or '96, he was convinced he was St George and that his coat of arms was a lion with a sword thrust through its body. While he seemed to recognise some of his men, he failed to recognise his wife or children. There were times when the king could predict the onset of an attack and he would order all weapons to be removed from the palace in the fears that he may hurt others, or himself.

In 1405, the king suddenly refused to bathe or change his clothes for five months because he was convinced his body was too brittle. Pope Pius II (1405–1464) wrote that he observed times when the king was sure he was made of glass and tried to protect himself so he would not break. He wore a special suit made of iron bars around his torso, and he wrapped his body in thick blankets and cushions. He was convinced that he would shatter if anyone came in contact with him, and he refused to be touched by even his most trusted servants.

The king would spend a great portion of his adult life believing that he could break into pieces at any moment.

Charles tried desperately to block his attacks with periods of prayer and pilgrimages to holy shrines. His doctors agreed that the king was suffering from an excess of black bile and attempted to remove it through frequent bleeding. A strict diet and rest were also prescribed. Several charlatans attempted to profit from the king's illness by promising a cure. During one attack, two men, claiming to be Augustan monks, provided powered pearls in the king's food, promising a swift recovery. Their attempts made no improvements, and they were eventually jailed and beheaded for treason.

Isabeau was known for her strength and support of her husband, and she brilliantly set up a regency council for the times when Charles was debilitated. Queen Isabeau had become one of the most prominent people in France as she held the country together in the hopes that her husband would recover for good.

Despite the fact that he'd taken a mistress and that the queen was rumoured to be having an affair with the king's brother, their relationship remained relatively solid. Throughout the king's illness, they were affectionate during his periods of lucidity, but she was wise enough to put distance between them when he fell into an attack.

His mental and physical disability prevented the king from conducting affairs of state, and civil war weakened the country. The people of France went from calling him 'Charles the Beloved' to 'Charles the Mad'. One chronicler noted: 'This caused great confusion and destroyed any equilibrium the government might have achieved.'[7]

Taking advantage of France's weakened state, the English king, Henry V (1386–1422), landed his army in 1415, claiming his stake to the French Crown. His brutal defeat of the French at the Battle of Agincourt (1415) resulted in his marriage to Charles's daughter, Catherine of Valois (1401–1437), in 1420 where both children were to rule France and England together.

Charles VI died in October of 1422 at the Hotel Saint-Pol. His son-in-law, Henry V, had died a few weeks prior, leaving an infant son who would reign as King Henry VI (1421–1471) of England.

Henry VI: Not the Warrior His Father Was

Henry VI was born at Windsor Castle on 6 December 1421. Henry would have big shoes to fill if he wanted to continue the legacy of his father. Henry V had been the epitome of medieval kingship. His stellar military successes in the Hundred Years' War made England one of the fiercest military powers in Europe.

Henry was a bright young boy who was described as robust and handsome. But he was also unlike his father in that bloodshed horrified him. Nonetheless, he took control of the government in 1437 at just 16 years old.

In 1445, Henry, aged 23, married 15-year-old Margaret of Anjou (1430–1482), but the match was unpopular as Margaret, unlike her husband, was very strong-willed and argumentative. Henry was known as a devoutly religious and kind man in his early reign and was said to have been 'unsteadfast of wit'[8]. He dressed in simple garments and didn't favour the elaborate clothes that were expected of a sovereign. He also continued to have a strong aversion to war. He had a simple mind and was honest, almost to a fault. He never purposely caused harm to anyone and encouraged others to share his love of religion. Instead of sports, he devoted his time to reading scripture and enjoyed attending public worship.

It took almost ten years for the queen to become pregnant, and when it usually would have been blamed on the woman, in this case, the blame lay with the king. It was said that he feared nakedness and had no understanding of what he was supposed to do in the marriage bed. Trusted attendants eventually had to join the couple in the bedroom for some coaching as an heir was desperately needed.

Henry quickly became an inconsistent ruler, and one commentator characterised his reign as a: 'dangerous compound of forcefulness and weakness'.[9]

The question of whether Henry could rule effectively came to a head in 1453 when he fell ill without warning. He showed signs of a sudden fright, where he went into a trance-like state and recognised no one, nor did he react to anyone. He sat with his eyes looking down, motionless, and ceased to speak. It was reported that he: 'fell by a sudden and accidental fright into such a weak state of health that for a whole year and a half, he had neither natural sense nor reason capable of carrying on the government, and neither physician nor medicine could cure that infirmity.'[10]

It was also noted that he: 'suddenly was taken and smitten with frenzy, and his wit and reason withdrawn'.[11]

Richard, Duke of York (1411–1460), was appointed the Lord Protector, but this did not sit well with Henry's queen, as she felt she should be governing the country.

After nine months, a deputation from the government went to visit the king but quickly learned there was no improvement in his condition: 'Entreaties, prayers, desire, lamentable cheer, exhortation, moving and stirring by all the wiles and means they could think of ... they could have no answer, word nor sign; and therefore, with a sorrowful heart, they returned to London.'[12]

In October 1453, Queen Margaret gave birth to a son, Edward of Lancaster (1453–1471)., Rumours quickly began to swirl, however, that the child was the son not of the king, but Edmund Beaufort, The Duke of Somerset (1406–1455), who was cousin to the Duke of York. The queen brought the baby to the king and pleaded with him to bless the child, but he only cast his eyes down and refused to look at him.

The king seemed to regain his lucidity several months later, and Prince Edward was brought to him again. He asked who the child was, and the queen informed him that he had a son. The king declared that Edward must have been fathered by the Holy Ghost, which only added to the doubts about the child's paternity. Nonetheless, he was pleased with the child, and his family was delighted to see that he had returned to his senses.

But the king's recovery was short-lived because in October of 1455, he again fell into a state of mental collapse and would not recover for a year. Chroniclers also noted that the king's personality had changed, and he continued to live in a weakened state of mind. Pope Pious II said the king was a: 'dolt and a fool, who is ruled instead of ruling'.

The queen urged Henry to counter the political aims of Richard of York, who still battled for control over the government as well as the succession to the throne. But the Yorkists usurped the king, forcing him to flee to Scotland, where he was imprisoned, and Richard's son Edward was declared the rightful king.

At the battle of Wakefield, the queen and the Lancastrians celebrated victory when they destroyed York's army, and Richard of York was killed in battle. Margaret of Anjou was reunited with Henry, who was brought to the second battle of St Albans (1461) roughly six weeks later with Yorkist ally, Richard Neville Earl of Warwick (1422–1471).

But Henry was reported to have been completely out of touch with reality. Historians have different takes on what went on, but several sources say he was found sitting under a tree, laughing, and talking to himself as the battle raged on. The Lancastrians defeated York again, this time taking the king with them. Henry was eventually returned to the throne in 1470, but his reign was short and ineffective.

Edward IV reclaimed the throne of England in 1471 and sent Henry to the Tower of London where he was imprisoned and eventually murdered by Richard, Duke of Gloucester.

The mental illness that affected Henry VI resulted in a total loss of reality and greatly compromised his ability to rule effectively. There is most likely a very strong genetic component to the illness, as we know that both Henry's mother and his grandfather suffered from psychosis, mania, and depression for years. The Abbott Weathampstead (1465) said in 1461 that Henry was: 'his mother's stupid offspring … a mild-spoken, pious king but half-witted in affairs of state'.[13]

The king's illness exhibited absent speech, immobility, catatonia, hallucinations, and the inability to function normally on a daily basis. These ailments, much like his grandfather's, are consistent with a modern-day diagnosis of schizophrenia. The disease has a very strong hereditary basis, and it's quite possible that Henry inherited a predisposition to a defective gene on his mother's side of the family. However, there are no known medical documents that exhibit the exact nature of his illness, so it's not certain that his illness was a mental one or if his symptoms evolved from a physical illness, such as syphilis or porphyria.

But it was not just the English and French monarchies that suffered from mental illness in the fifteenth century. Not far, in the warmer climate of Spain, lived another ruling family that was also afflicted.[14]

Chapter Five

The House of Aviz, Trastamara and the Sad Story of Juana the Mad

Isabella I of Castile remains among the most powerful women in the Middle Ages. From 1474 until her death in 1504, she ruled as queen of Castile alongside her husband, King Ferdinand II of Aragon. The power couple were referred to as the first monarchs to be king and queen of Spain alongside one another.

Isabella was the driving force behind the Alhambra Decree (1492), which ordered the mass expulsion of Muslims and Jews from Spain. The decree accused Jews of trying to pervert the Catholic faith and lead Christians from their duty and beliefs. The Jewish population of Spain was given four months to convert to Christianity or be banished from the country. The punishment for anyone who did not convert or flee was execution. Isabella and Ferdinand were also responsible for the deaths of thousands during the Spanish Inquisition (1478–1834).

From what we understand, Isabella suffered no mental illness and was able to govern her empire with an intelligence and fierceness that would have her long remembered throughout history. However, her mother, and daughter, were not so lucky. Mental illness often skips generations, and in the case of the Spanish queens of Europe, we see great evidence of this.

The mother of Isabella I of Castile suffered from mental illness for the better portion of her life, and we must strongly consider that it may have been due to her parents being uncle and half-niece.

Isabella of Portugal (1428–1496) was the daughter of John, Constable of Portugal (1400–1442). In 1424, he married Isabel of Braganza (1402–1466), the daughter of his half-brother, Alfonso

(1377–1461). The couple went on to have three children, Isabella being one of two daughters.

Isabella belonged to the House of Aviz (1383–1580), a Portuguese dynasty that thrived during the early years of the Renaissance. The House of Aviz was founded by King John I of Portugal (1357–1433), Isabella's grandfather. The monarchs of the House of Aviz would rule Portugal through the Age of Discovery following the creation of the Portuguese empire (1415).

In 1445, Isabella became the second wife of John II of Castile (1405–1454). During her marriage, Isabella was said to be a possessive, and jealous wife who was also violent at times. In 1450 she became pregnant with the couple's first daughter, the future Isabella I of Castile. When sent into confinement towards the end of her pregnancy, which was common practice for royals, she refused to see or speak to anyone except her husband.

When a queen or woman of nobility reached the end of her pregnancy, she would go into confinement or 'lying in'. After several prayers from clergy members, a queen was confined to her private rooms and kept from the public eye. Lying in meant the rooms being closed off and devoid of sunlight. Men were forbidden from entering, and the woman could only be tended to by other women. With the exception of one small window, the rest of the windows would be covered with dark tapestries and kept shut. Medieval physicians believed that too much sunlight was detrimental to pregnant women's eyes. The purpose of lying in was to keep the queen calm and rested before the treacherous ordeal of childbirth. The room was, in a sense, designed to be like the womb. It was a dark, warm, and quiet atmosphere. And certainly, intentions were good, but it's easy to imagine that one might go stir-crazy in a setting like this – especially when forced to remain there for several weeks.

However, for Isabella of Portugal, her symptoms of solitude didn't end after the birth of her daughter. In fact, they worsened. She continued to keep herself shut away and fell into a deep postpartum depression. She became what many called a 'nervous invalid'. She often stared into nothing for hours at a time, not moving or talking, and appeared almost statue-like. The only person she showed any emotion to was her husband, and it was often an unpleasant encounter as she easily went into hysterics.

In 1453, the pattern of postpartum depression repeated itself after the birth of Isabella's son, Alfonso, Prince of Asturias (1453–1468). John II of Castile died a year later, and she spent the remainder of her life in exile at Arevalo Castle. When her two children moved on to further their political careers, Isabella sank deeper into melancholy. We must assume that being isolated in a desolate castle, widowed and away from her children, would have only made her mental health suffer even more. Her servants reported that along with growing physically aggressive towards them, Isabella eventually lost all recognition of people. She failed to remember who she was and began to talk to herself. She was often seen wandering the castle, yelling at imaginary enemies, whom she claimed were voices of the long deceased.

Isabella of Portugal died in 1496 at the age of 67, well past the life expectancy of a fifteenth-century woman. Perhaps part of the reason she lived as long as she did was because she was confined and probably kept safe from plague and other maladies of the time. But if we consider the fact that she lived a life of solace and melancholy for over forty years, we can perhaps conclude that she most likely died as a result of the mental exhaustion her condition caused her.

From the accomplishments of Isabella's daughter, Isabella I of Castile, we can assume that she most likely avoided the unhappiness that plagued her mother for so many years. But Isabella's life was not an easy one.

When she was born, she was second in line to the throne after her half-brother, Henry IV of Castile (1425–1474). Henry ascended the throne when their father died, and Isabella and her younger brother Alfonso were left in his care. Isabella, along with her mother and brother, were moved to live in a castle in Arevalo.

Life was not easy for her, as the conditions at the castle were incredibly poor, and there was a shortage of funds. Isabella's father made it clear in his will that his children be kept financially sound, but King Henry did not comply – probably because he wanted to keep his half-siblings under his control.

When the king and his wife were expecting their first child, both Isabella and her brother were called to court in Segovia, where Isabella became part of the queen's household. Her living conditions were much improved. Besides having plenty to eat and lots of clothing, she found herself living in a place that was elaborately decorated with silver and gold.

Isabella was educated extensively in writing, reading, grammar, mathematics, chess, embroidery, music, and dancing. She was also given a rigorous religious education. While she enjoyed a pleasant lifestyle, she was forbidden from leaving Segovia.

The story of Isabella's betrothals and marriage was a long and complicated one. At the age of 6, she was betrothed to the younger son of John II of Navarre (1398–1479). But this arrangement did not last. In 1465, there was talk of a marriage between Isabella and Afonso V of Portugal (1432–1481). But Isabella did not favour the marriage, and she refused.

King Henry IV was inept at ruling; a civil war broke out in Castile and he needed a way to restore peace in his kingdom. Isabella was then betrothed to Pedro Giron Acuna Pacheco (1423–1466), the brother of the king's greatest friend. However, Pedro died on his way to meet her.

Afonso V of Portugal was still an option according to King Henry, but again Isabella refused. She made a promise to marry her very first betrothed, Ferdinand of Aragon. His father, John of Aragon (1350–1396), negotiated with the couple regarding a secret marriage. A formal betrothal was announced in October 1469. However, Isabella and Ferdinand were second cousins and stood within the degrees of consanguinity.

Early canon law prohibited anyone more closely related than seventh cousins from marriage. This ban on cousin marriage weakened the structures of kinship that defined many European populations. With the choice of non-related spouses narrowing, the nobility struggled to find partners to wed. Many of those who wished to marry had to disobey the laws of the church or find another spouse. Even those who unintentionally married within the family would often find their marriage annulled by the church.

During the eleventh and twelfth centuries however, things began to change. The church's strict laws on marriage were a hardship for those who wanted to carry on family lineage. Remember that the Catholic Church was not without corruption in the highest offices, where clergy often lived extravagant lifestyles. As part of a sort of 'fundraising scheme', the forgiveness of sins or a papal dispensation could easily be bought for the right price by the nobility. In 1215, a change to canon law would now allow the degree of consanguinity to fourth cousins unless a papal dispensation, or exemption, was granted.

For Ferdinand and Isabella, this meant a papal bull would be needed. One was given, authorising them to marry and make the marriage legal. They married in October of 1469 in the city of Valladolid.

Isabella's reign was off to a rough start with several plots against her life, yet she prevailed and led her country fearlessly. She also seemingly escaped the hell of mental illness that had afflicted her mother. The same fortitude that Queen Isabella of Castile possessed can not be said for her daughter, Juana of Castile, of the House of Trástamara.

The House of Trástamara was a lineage of rulers from both the Castilian and Aragonese thrones. Often historically referred to as 'Juana the Mad', Juana of Castile was born in 1479. While she was in the care of her wet nurse, Juana, like her brothers and sisters, was kept close to her parents. Her father was attentive, often gifted her with dolls to play with, and gave her sweets such as lemon blossoms. She was said to be a lovely child who grew into a great beauty, sporting the same fair complexion and auburn hair as her mother. As with her sisters, Juana grew up under the strict tutelage of their mother. She knew at a young age that her purpose in life was to marry and birth many sons in the name of God.

Isabella, considered to be one of the most educated women in Europe, was adamant that her children got a proper education, which included music, history, literature, language and most importantly, Catholicism. Her daughters were all needed to cement useful alliances with foreign countries to benefit Spain.

Isabella herself was a fervent Catholic. When she came to the throne, Islamic rule had been in place for over 700 years in many regions of Spain. As we know, the new Catholic queen, along with her husband, would soon change that. She was confident and ruled with a precise strategy that soon made her a large influence on Rome. After gaining tremendous favour with the Pope, Isabella was determined to spread Catholicism not only throughout her immediate family, but also her kingdom.

Perhaps Juana's first brush with grief was when she was 11 years old. Her older sister Isabella (1470–1498) lost her husband in a riding accident. She was utterly devastated, and Juana witnessed first-hand the trauma of her grief.

Queen Isabella's teachings on the Catholic faith did not sit well with her 16-year-old daughter. Juana was in the middle of teenage rebellion, preferring hunting and hawking to learning about religion – her scepticism enraged her mother. It's possible that Juana may have been interested in Protestantism, but either way, the queen would not tolerate heresy in any form. And it would seem she cared more about 'fixing' Juana's wayward thinking than she did about her life. But we must remember that this was a different time with a different way of thinking, especially when it came to fervent Catholics.

Isabella used a method of torture known as *la cuerda* in an attempt to correct Juana (not surprising, as *la cuerda* was used throughout the Spanish Inquisition, with which Queen Isabella was widely associated). In this form of ruthlessness, the hands of the victim would be tied behind their back, and they would be hung from the ceiling by their arms. The object was to cause the shoulders to pull out of their sockets, causing tremendous pain and the hope of a confession. Isabella took it a step further when she added weights to her daughter's feet. While she firmly believed she was saving her daughter's soul, Juana refused to admit to heresy or any other wrongdoing.

As with most royal daughters of the medieval period, Juana was expected to make a proper wife for the political advancements of her family and country. At age 16, she was betrothed to 17-year-old Philip of Burgundy (1478–1506), or Philip the Handsome, as he was commonly known. Born in 1478, Philip was the oldest son of Maximillian I, Holy Roman Emperor (1459–1519), and Mary of Burgundy (1457–1482). Philip's fair-coloured hair and stunning blue eyes would make it easy for Juana to fall in love with him.

After being married by proxy, travel arrangements were made, and Isabella ensured that her daughter would be sent off in style with expensive jewels and clothes. She was also sent with plenty of cattle and chickens so that she would never go hungry. Juana boarded a ship at the point of Laredo and left her mother, who prayed for her safety. It was a rough journey, and while some of her belongings got misplaced, Juana eventually made it to Burgundy. When she arrived, however, Philip was in Germany, and it would be almost a month before she would meet him.

Many betrothed couples of the time had little or no attraction to one another, but this was far from the case with Juana and Philip. Juana was 17, healthy and beautiful. Her auburn hair, deep blue eyes, and pouty mouth immediately caught Philip's attention. They were due to marry on 20 October 1496, but when Philip saw her, he was so smitten with Juana that he asked a priest to bless their marriage before the ceremony so he could bed her properly. It was love at first sight for them both, and they eagerly made their way to the royal bed chamber as soon as possible.

While the passion was immediate, it seemed that Philip was also eager to assert political dominance over his wife, gradually causing her to feel demoralised, which only added to the sadness of what her life would become. Philip demanded she give him control of the running of her household and took over her finances, refusing to give her the money allotted to her as part of the marital agreement. Juana soon found herself with no money and unable even to afford to pay her servants, many of whom began to stray. Because she was young and inexperienced, she wasn't sure how to handle Philip's possessiveness, and all she felt for him was lust.

Philip appointed his old governess, Madame de Hallewin, to be Juana's key lady-in-waiting. This was a woman who greatly intimidated her and often reduced her to tears. Juana began to feel homesick and would often retreat to her rooms to cry. Aside from the obvious beginning of their marital discord, the couple appeared relatively happy in public. Philip was keen on presenting his wife with elaborate gifts, such as necklaces, saddles, and pictures.

Luckily for Juana, she bore children easily. Her firstborn was a girl named Eleanor (1498–1558). However, she was not so lucky in that she birthed a daughter and not a son. Philip expected his wife to pay for the baby's attendants herself because he had no interest in funding a daughter, stating: 'When God grants us with a son, I will provide.'

Thankfully, Juana gave birth to a son in 1500, whom they named Charles. A display of fireworks filled the sky, and Philip gave his wife an emerald necklace. In 1501, another daughter named Isabella was born.

When Juana's brother, Juan (1478–1497), passed, Philip took a keen interest in inheriting her parent's kingdom. Now that there was no longer a male heir in the way, he had the motive to be more aggressive. He overlooked the fact that Juana was now heir and figured that what was hers was his.

The couple visited Spain in 1502, but before they arrived, Isabella heard rumours that Juana was still distancing herself from the Catholic faith and it worried her greatly. To add to her concern, she immediately noticed that something was amiss when the couple arrived. She noticed Philip's eagerness to acquire Juana's lands. But while in Spain, Juana was a queen in her own right and Isabella felt compelled to protect her. Regardless of (or perhaps because of) Philip's general cruelty towards Juana, she became pregnant again. Isabella pleaded with her to stay in Spain so she could counsel her on governing, but Philip had no interest in remaining in Spain, so he left his wife – pregnant with their fourth child – in Spain. He knew she was in no condition to travel and yet had no interest in waiting for her to deliver her baby.

In 1503, another boy, Ferdinand (1503–1564), was born. Philip wanted his wife back with him in Burgundy, but Isabella urged her daughter to consider staying in Spain longer. Despite being torn, Juana chose to return to her husband. When her mother tried again to persuade her to stay, Juana became hysterical. This was the first incidence of a behaviour with which she would soon become synonymous.

Juana then refused to eat, talk, or sleep. She stood in the pouring rain, trying desperately to convince a ship's captain to return her to Burgundy that night, as she did not want to wait until May 1504 to return to her husband. She wanted to return to the country she now thought of as home and to the man she loved.

Her reunion with Philip was not what she expected. He had a wandering eye and had begun to fancy other women of the court. This did not sit well with Juana, who, much like her grandmother, had a jealous streak which caused her to fly into a rage over her husband's behaviour. She felt terribly betrayed by her husband's misplaced passion. She soon discovered that her husband had a mistress and had been unfaithful. She once again flew into a jealous rage. Taking a pair of scissors, she cut off the woman's hair and then proceeded to stab her in the face.

In desperation, Juana attempted to win back her husband's affections by using 'love potions'. When this failed, she accused him of having an affair with every woman at court; she soon developed a reputation for mental instability, which would forever be used against her. The couple argued fervently, and Juana began to fall into a depression. Philip grew tired of his wife's outbursts and chose to ignore her when things got heated. He also kept detailed reports on her behaviour and sent letters to her parents in Spain to humiliate her.

When Isabella fell ill in 1504, Juana travelled to see her. Isabella had been sick with high fevers and dropsy. Juana was so distraught that her mother was sick that she refused to eat or sleep. But soon, they began to argue as well, and Juana wanted to return home to Philip once again.

Because travelling through France would have been too dangerous at the time as the two countries were at war, Juana's servants wanted to return by sea. Juana was adamant they travelled by foot and went into an even deeper rage when her horses were put away in their stalls, and she proceeded to stay outside near the stables in desperation to free them.

While Isabella lay dying, she continued receiving letters from her son-in-law about Juana's behaviour. Isabella worried about the fate of Castile if it was left to her unstable daughter and her domineering husband. She and Ferdinand had worked their entire lives together as king and queen, but they had always respected each other's lands and she feared Philip would not be so understanding. Isabella was convinced that Juana had inherited her grandmother's mental instability, and so she put a clause in her will stating that Juana, as an heiress to her lands: 'may be absent from them or, after having come to them and stayed in them for some time, may be unable to reign and govern. If such were the case, it would be necessary to provide that the government should be nevertheless carried on.'[1]

It's worth considering if Isabella was somehow trying to pave the way for her daughter's exclusion, along with the fact that she wanted Philip to have nothing to do with Castile. What she clearly meant in her clause by 'might not be able to govern' was that Philip may do everything in his power to prevent his wife from governing. Isabella included in her clause that Ferdinand should rule Castile until Prince Charles was of age and that Juana and Philip must obey him in all things as 'good and obedient children and listen to his advice on all matters'.[2]

After a lengthy illness, on 24 November 1504, Isabella I of Castile passed away, and Juana was now Queen Regent of Castile. Juana's marriage to Philip was not getting any better. They argued constantly, and some witnesses say it became physical. Philip was becoming tyrannical, and he locked Juana in her rooms and sent her beloved Moorish servants back to Spain. He dismissed several of her ladies and tried to keep her secluded.

Publicly, Ferdinand was respectful that Castile was his daughter's land, but what he intended was to maintain control himself, even if that meant he had to abandon her. Juana was 26 years old and would soon have both her father and her husband plotting against her. Philip sent a letter to Ferdinand stating that Juana claimed she wanted her husband to handle her lands and rule in her place. But this was far from the truth; she was desperate to return to Spain and to her people. To gain control, both men would soon elaborate on the growing rumours that Juana was not of sound mind.

Juana always appeared well-behaved in public, which cast doubt on Philip's claims that his wife was losing her mind. When the couple visited Brussels in 1505, Juana sat through a joust and banquet with all the grace of a queen. The Venetian Ambassador said that Juana: 'looked very well ... her being that of a sensible and discreet woman'.[3]

Although Philip treated his wife horribly throughout their marriage, the couple still had a passion for each other. Juana refused to accept Philip's infidelities and remained jealous of any woman that even looked at him. She also became pregnant with their fifth child and gave birth to another daughter in 1505 before they prepared to go to Spain. She was adamant that her husband had no female attendants on this journey because she was convinced he would try to bed all of them. She went into a terrible rage while arguing with her husband, insisting that this be carried forth. Unfortunately, her actions only gave Philip's words more validity when he ranted about her insanity.

The start of 1505 would mark the beginning of Juana's total betrayal. Her father had secured a regency over Castile, and he presented evidence to the council that his daughter was unfit to rule.

He also presented them with Isabella's clause, and the council quickly agreed that Juana was inept at governing. Her 'infirmity' was now well publicised, and Ferdinand was determined to deal with Castile and its politics.

In addition to her father plotting against her, Philip was also busy with his own plans. He had negotiated with France, building up his own support to rule Castile. He also claimed that he was willing to ally with Ferdinand as long as he could declare Juana insane and keep her locked away. They eventually agreed to a three-way rule, but either way, Juana's lands would never be hers.

Philip and Juana set sail for Castile in January of 1506 with a fleet of ships. They hit fierce weather that caused some of their ships to struggle to stay afloat. Their ship was blown off course and ended up in Weymouth at Dorset, England. There they were rescued by Henry VII's men, who had been sent when he heard of the unplanned landing. Philip was eager to meet the king, so he set off immediately, leaving his wife in Dorset. Philip enjoyed food and entertainment in the company of the English king. Juana eventually made it to Windsor to meet her husband and was thrilled to see her sister, Katherine of Aragon (1485–1436), daughter-in-law of the king; Philip, however, seemed reluctant to let Henry meet Juana. Was it because he had told him how twisted she was mentally, and if she appeared calm, Henry might be suspicious? Philip made sure his wife's visits with the king were short, so it's possible he didn't want to jeopardise his plans. To earn support for the lands of Castile, everyone must see how unfit Juana was. The couple stayed in England until April, but Philip managed to keep Juana away from the king almost the entire time.

On 26 April 1506, they docked in Coruna, and Juana noticed that she didn't have the support she was hoping for. All her ladies were now chosen by her husband, her officials were bribed by him, and he also did his best to keep her from seeing her father. Nevertheless, Juana waited patiently to see Fernando as she didn't want to upset him. This played into Philip's aim of keeping her away from as many people as possible for the same reason that he had tried to keep her from King Henry of England. Because she seemed to flutter between periods of lucidity and insanity, Philip was terrified that people might see her as perfectly normal.

Philip kept his wife content by being an attentive and passionate lover, and because Juana was so in love with him, she tried her best to keep any arguments to a minimum. She was also fearful that he would continue to take her from her lands and so she made love to her husband with the same passion they shared from day one.

During this time, Ferdinand and Philip were growing closer and realised their best option for power was for Ferdinand to ignore his daughter and make no immediate attempts to see her. Ferdinand left Castile in Philip's hands for the time being, excluding his daughter, who was the only rightful heir. They also went out of their way to ensure Juana had no supporters.

Juana was terrified and helpless about what to do as her husband continued to dominate her every move and assert himself over her. Slowly, Ferdinand grew suspicious that maybe his son-in-law didn't have the best of intentions. He began to see that Philip was greedy and wanted Castile for himself and would not have agreed to anything if he knew this were the case. Ferdinand made a declaration before his public notary that he still had all authority over Castile.

But still, no matter how determined she was to see him, Philip kept Juana from seeing her father. One day during a gentle ride on her horse, Juana suddenly took off at a gallop as she tried to find her father. But she was subdued by Philip's soldiers and went willingly when they caught her. It is not known whether Ferdinand knew of this attempt. But he did instruct Philip to: 'cultivate a better understanding with the queen, his wife, whose health depended upon gentle measures being used'.[4]

He also told Philip he would not stand for her being incarcerated in any way, despite Philip repeatedly telling him that she was insane. Ferdinand then left for Italy on business.

In September 1506, Philip and Juana travelled to the city of Burgos, and Philip became ill. He was convinced he had simply overindulged in food and drink, but a fever quickly developed.

Despite Philip's cruel treatment of Juana throughout their marriage, she behaved as a dutiful and caring wife should. She truly valued the Catholic sanctity of marriage, even if she had strayed from her faith. She was also five months pregnant but put all her comfort aside to care for her husband, and never left his side.

On 25 September, Philip died of what is believed to be typhoid fever. Because the death was swift, many believed that he may have been poisoned by Juana's father in yet another attempt to compete for the crown of Castile.

With her husband dead and her father in Italy, Juana must have felt truly alone and unsure of how to proceed regarding her lands. She wanted to take control of what was hers, but the Archbishop of Toledo (1472–1545), who had been her mother's confessor, questioned her devotion to the Catholic faith and saw her as incapable of ruling. Perhaps he was right in some ways, as she had depleted finances and few supporters. Juana also had a strong maternal instinct to protect her eldest son's inheritance. Charles was 6 and was being raised by Philip's sister with Burgundy tradition, not Spanish. Charles hardly knew his mother, as his only memory of her may have been when she left him in the care of others as an infant.

It was after the death of her husband that Juana's madness truly began to surface. She was so distraught over his passing that she refused to leave his side, even after death. Perhaps to ease her pain, she ordered that his coffin be opened on more than one occasion so she could see him. In her grief, she would not only stare at her husband's corpse, but kissed his cold lips and held him in her arms.

She refused to see anyone or sign anything until the end of the year. Just before Christmas 1506, Juana ordered that her husband's coffin be brought from the Monastery of Mira Flores to Granada, where she wished to bury him. She wanted his place in Spanish history to be assured, and she wanted him to have the honour of being buried as a king with a male heir.

The journey to Granada from Burgos was over 400 miles and would have taken at least a week. Despite being eight months pregnant, Juana went on the journey with several monks, staying close to her husband's body. She insisted that they travel only at night, as she didn't want any women to see her husband's beauty, for she felt another woman may feel desire for him, even after days of being deceased. Because of her fear that other women may view her husband, she would only stop and rest at monasteries as she felt that even the nuns might find themselves attracted to Philip.

Juana went into labour during the trip and gave birth in the town of Torquemada before resuming the journey. When she went into labour, she refused the help of a midwife and instead gave birth by herself to her sixth child, a daughter named Catalina (1507–1578).

Philip was eventually brought to Granada, and Juana returned to Castile. Her father was also returning to Castile to deal with the turmoil. He said he would: 'give up my own comforts and undergo all the labour of assisting Juana and her kingdoms'.[5]

At first, Juana tried to rule Castile by herself. However, the odds were not in her favour when the country was hit with a poor harvest, and plague had begun to work its way through the kingdom. As fate would have it, her father arrived back in Castile as the plague was on its way out. He also arrived in time for a fresh, thriving harvest. The people of Castile saw this as an intervention of the Lord and felt it was God's way of saying he approved of Ferdinand as a ruler. He was greeted warmly by the people.

He also returned, making it seem like he was the devoted father coming to care for his daughter, but we know by now he had ulterior motives. He wanted Castile for himself and stated that his daughter was: 'so overcome by the death of Philip that she couldn't rule. She suffered a blow which caused unspeakable affliction, rendering her incapable.'[6]

She went into seclusion, filled with despair with her country falling apart, and Ferdinand played on her grief to his benefit. In a letter to a Spanish Adversary, he said:

> My daughter was still carrying with her the corpse of King Philip, her late husband. Before I arrived, they could never persuade her to bury him. Even with my arrival, she said she does not wish the said corpse to be buried. On account of her health and in order to content her, I do not contradict her in anything … but I shall endeavour to persuade her by degrees to permit the corpse to be buried.[7]

Perhaps in a moment of sanity, Juana submitted to her father's wishes. She agreed to let him do whatever he thought necessary. He also took over the finances and her household. She withdrew even more and suggested that her three-year-old son, Fernando, was better off with his grandfather.

In September of 1509, Ferdinand received more news about his daughter. She had entered a period of odd behaviour and was like a young, feeble child. She refused to eat or drink for days and was known to throw tantrums. She also sank deeper into her religious indifference. Ferdinand wished his daughter to remain in Tordesillas so she couldn't try to return to her husband's corpse. She was kept comfortable in the Royal Monastery of Santa Clara. She had a pleasant view and most of her personal belongings with her. Her daughter Catalina was also allowed to stay with her, which gave her great comfort.

Ferdinand would only visit his daughter twice before falling ill in January 1516. While travelling, he died of an unknown cause, leaving some of his lands to his grandson Fernando, and some to Juana. It would be years before Juana was informed that her father had passed away; because she could not rule, her son Charles governed at 16 as he would be the heir to Castile and Aragon should Juana pass away.

Ambassadors in Venetia gave Charles reports of his mother's condition. 'She expects her husband to come to life again. She says his resurrection will take place at the end of ten years.'[8]

Though her son, Charles, did visit Juana, he never improved her living conditions. She was still isolated and withdrawn from others, and by the time she was 37, she had already spent seven years in Tordesillas under the watch of her father's appointee, Mosen Ferrer. She had now been moved to only two small rooms, and other than having an occasional visitor, she spent her time eating, sleeping, talking with her daughter, and reading. Juana loved to read and had over 300 books on religion, including missals and a Book of Hours. She also had several medical treatises on melancholy.

When Juana grew frustrated, she would revert to refusing all food and cease to sleep; she was also known to physically attack some of her servants. But then news got out that Ferrer was mistreating her. The townspeople grew irate at these rumours and began to riot. Several priests were sent to 'heal the queen'. Neither Charles nor Cardinal Cisneros (1436–1517) liked the chaos, and Ferrer was ordered away from Juana. He denied treating her badly and said it was her fault, but there was physical evidence that he was beating her.

Charles made no attempt to visit his ill mother and left everything in the care of Cardinal Cisneros. He said: 'while she is to be treated well, she be so well guarded and watched that if any persons should endeavour to counteract any good intentions, they shall be prevented from doing so. In this respect, great vigilance is necessary.'[9]

Ferrer was replaced by the Marquis of Denia and his wife, both of whom supported Charles's cause. Denia treated Juana far worse than Ferrer had. Denia stopped Juana from visiting the convent, where she had found comfort in the sisters. He claimed that she pestered him too much, and he continued to make excuses about it being inconvenient, or that too much disease was in the air. Part of this need to keep her locked away may have been at the request of Charles. Much like her husband, he did not want Juana to appear in public in case it was on a day when she was lucid. Charles ordered that Denia not write or speak of the queen to anyone except him.

If Juana asked to meet with nobles, Denia denied her, stating again that there was too much disease in the air and the journey was too far for anyone to make. He also denied her medical care. At one point, she was suffering from a terrible toothache but was denied a doctor because 'everyone was unwell because of the weather'. At one point, Juana had such a high fever that she found herself shaking for days and begged for a doctor, but again this was denied.

When asked of her health, Denia told Charles, 'She lives in her room, goes to bed and gets up and dines every second day'.[10]

Charles seemed to care more for his teenage sister, Catalina, and told her she may leave whenever she saw fit, but she refused to leave her ailing mother. Charles's suggestion put Juana in a state of paranoia, and she became afraid to let Catalina out of her sight. She promised that if her daughter were taken away, she would kill herself with a knife or by jumping out a window. When Catalina came of age and had to leave to get married, her mother was broken with grief and stood in the doorway through which her daughter had departed for twenty-four hours after she left. She then shut herself away for two days.

Charles had declared himself king and Holy Roman Emperor. However, his rise to the throne was not without its problems. He was seen as inexperienced as a king, and many Spaniards disagreed with his rule. They felt he might focus on inheriting lands from the Holy Roman Emperor, Maximillian (1459–1519). Riots against Charles followed, and as the rebellion spread into northern Spain, attempts were made to return Juana to her place as the rightful queen.

In August of 1520, a group of officials demanded to see her. They told her that her father had been dead for years and that Castile was again in turmoil. Many people were angered over Charles's abuse of power and told Juana she was the only one who could save them. These rebels, or Comuneros, were desperate to get Juana ready to rule. She asked for political counsel to be sent to her, but Tordesillas soon fell under rebel control.

They made their way into the castle and immediately asked Denia and his wife to leave. Denia begged the queen to intercept, but she only said to 'leave her alone and not to speak with her'.[11]

Juana was gracious enough to meet with the rebels over the next few months and listen to their stories of unrest. They encouraged her to have confidence in herself that she could govern on her own. All she had to do was sign a proclamation. But Juana was not persuaded that easily. She said she loved her people but was sorry she would not sign anything. She informed the rebels that she was still filled with grief over her father's death and that her heart needed to heal. She told the rebels that she often felt unwell and tired; inwardly, she wasn't sure she totally trusted them.

When Charles's army eventually took back control, Juana showed only loyalty towards her son. Sadly, Charles proved he wasn't as devoted to her. He refused to let anyone see her and Denia was reinstated. Juana soon fell back into her old routines of refusing to eat or change her clothes. Writing to Charles, Denia claimed this was due to the attention she had received during the revolt, and that she had become 'so spoiled and haughty that there is no man who has not had great difficulty with her. In truth, if Your Majesty would apply the torture, it would in many respects be a service and a good thing, rendered to God and to Her Highness.'[12]

We are not sure exactly what Denia meant by torture, but we do know that Charles approved the use of whips and the rack on his mother if she got out of control.

Catalina wrote to her brother on her mother's behalf:

> Your Majesty ought, for the love of God, to provide that
> if the queen, my Lady, wishes to go to the large room to
> refresh herself, she not be prevented from doing so. They
> direct the woman not to let her go to the large room or to
> the corridors. But they lock her up in her chamber where
> no other light enters except by candlelight, and there is
> no room where she could retire from that chamber.[13]

Charles ignored his sister's pleas.

In 1543, Juana was visited by several of her grandchildren, which pleased her greatly. Other than a few visits, Juana probably passed her time reading, but she soon lost the ability to feed, bathe, or clothe herself. She grew paranoid and was certain the sisters who cared for her were now her sworn enemies or witches. She could hardly stand to hear the voices of Denia and his wife, which surely didn't help her slow deterioration.

Juana died in 1555 at the age of 75. She was a frail woman who spent her last weeks lying in bed, too weak to move or to have her soiled bed linens changed. She was buried alongside Philip and given the honours of a queen.

Juana of Castile led a sad life plagued by severe mental illness. Physicians today believe she may have suffered from not only depression, but also schizophrenia and bipolar disorder. Whether or not we have an accurate diagnosis, we do know that Juana was another example of a young and beautiful woman who was placed in a position of power, despite her afflictions in life.

Nonetheless, a complex spider web would soon develop in her family as cousins married cousins. The past would reach down to tickle the present and slowly shape the future of what would be the Habsburg Monarchy, which will discover in a later chapter.

Queen Katherine and Her Failed Pregnancies

If we consider Juana's sister, Katherine of Aragon, there are no stories of mental illness plaguing her. Katherine, the first wife of England's Henry VIII, was a beloved queen and fierce warrior like her mother. But Katherine could not fulfil the one duty expected of all European monarchs: to produce a male heir.

Katherine married Henry VIII in June of 1509, and the couple fell very much in love. Katherine was beautiful, with the same stunning red hair shared by her mother and sister. Henry was enthralled by his new Queen and eager to get to work on carrying on the Tudor dynasty. and in November of that same year, Katherine's first pregnancy was announced to the public, and Henry's Kingdom rejoiced. However, in late January of the following year, Katherine went into labour prematurely, giving birth to a stillborn daughter, which shook Katherine to her core. She had wanted so very much to give the king and the people of England a healthy prince. Henry and Katherine wasted no time in their attempts to secure the monarchy, and in May of 1510, Katherine was pregnant again. Her pregnancy was unremarkable, and she carried the baby to term.

On New Year's Day, in the early hours of 1511, Katherine had a baby boy. The announcement to court stated that:

'The queen has delivered of a Prince to the great gladness of the realm.'

The child, called Henry after his father, was celebrated with bonfires in London. Tragically, only fifty-two days later, the new prince. Devastated by the loss, Henry planned a lavish funeral for the prince at Westminster Abbey.

It would be over two years before Katherine of Aragon would give birth again. Katherine may have gone into labour before her due date, but all we know is that this new prince of England was either born deceased or died shortly afterwards. A little over a year later, in November of 1514, yet another stillborn son was delivered. The baby was seven or eight months' gestation, and his death was grieved throughout court.

In February of 1516, Katherine and Henry would welcome a daughter, whom they called Mary. She would be the couple's only surviving child and would later reign as Queen Mary I of England. In November 1518, Katherine yet again gave birth to a nearly full-term child, a daughter, also stillborn. This would be Katherine's last pregnancy. Out of six pregnancies, five of them ended in the death of the child.

There have been many speculations as to why Katherine lost so many children. While it wasn't terribly unusual during the time to lose a pregnancy, five in just nine years, was a lot. Some reports say that Henry was infertile, but through mistresses and other wives, he had several children. Others say that Katherine was under such great pressure to produce a son that it caused only stress, which in turn, caused the miscarriages.

But we also must consider that Katherine's parents were cousins, which may have increased the risk of infant death in the family. Clearly, Katherine had no problems conceiving. It was carrying a healthy baby to term that plagued her. Given that her parents did share a blood relation, it is entirely possible that this contributed to her frequent delivery of stillborn babies. A 1999 study posted in the The National Library of Medicine indicates that even being second cousins can increase neonatal death and infant mortality. Even if Katherine herself didn't practice inbreeding, she was the result of royal intermarriage.

If we step ahead a generation to Katherine's only living daughter, Mary, we can see some correlation in her regarding both mental instability and infertility. While it's not easy to determine how much of a factor her grandparent's blood relation was in her life, I feel it is well worth mentioning.

Chapter Six

The House of Tudor, Stewart, James V of Scotland and the Three Troubled Queens

Mary Tudor was born in February 1516 and would be the only surviving child of King Henry VIII and Katherine of Aragon. Throughout history Mary is often recorded as a vile and ruthless woman. While she was responsible for the persecution of Protestants during her reign, I must wonder if some of her behaviour was, at least in part, due to some kind of mental struggle.

While she wasn't the long-awaited prince of Henry and Katherine, she was still greatly loved by her parents during early childhood. Inheriting red hair from both her parents, Mary was a delightful child who was the apple of her father's eye. She was highly educated and brought up as a fervent Catholic like her mother and grandmother.

While princes became kings, princesses were used as political pawns to secure the throne. Mary was betrothed twice – the first time at the age of two– but both betrothals ended when she was still a child. It seemed as if these two failed betrothals were an indication of how unfortunate Mary's life would be. Once the doted-on princess, Mary's childhood would soon take a turn for the worse.

In 1526, after over fifteen years without a male heir, Mary's father Henry was becoming frustrated, and the queen's childbearing years seemed to be coming to an end.

Young Mary would watch in horror as her father ended his marriage to her mother with the promise that his new queen, Anne Boleyn (1507–1536), would give him a much-desired son. Henry declared that his marriage to Katherine had been no marriage at all, and that Princess Mary was therefore a bastard.

There was certainly no love lost between Mary and her new stepmother. She saw Anne as no more than the woman who had ruined her parents' marriage and was intent on stealing her mother's crown.

In the summer of 1529, Henry sent Katherine away to Kimbolton House in Cambridgeshire. Mary would never see her mother again. Her beloved father, whom she adored, had managed to turn her life upside down. In addition to banishing her mother from court, he also broke with the Catholic Church that Mary loved so much, to marry Anne Boleyn.

Mary would not become queen of England until 1553 and would spend decades in turmoil to get there. Her mother died in 1536, alone and without any comfort save her only servant. Mary's world fell apart when she learned her mother had died, and she also had to endure four more of her father's wives after Anne Boleyn was executed on charges of adultery.

Mary very much favoured her father's third wife, Jane Seymour (1508–1537), who was kind and did her best to convince Henry to let Mary back into her life. But Jane died in childbirth, leaving Henry a widow and Mary the half-sister to Edward, the next king of England. Mary was saddened by Jane's death and most likely viewed it as yet another loss in her life.

She would also watch in disgust as her father married twice more, with the fifth wife being closer to Mary's age than her father's. But Mary did have a fondness for her father's sixth wife, Katherine Parr (1512–1548). Katherine was kind and motherly and took both Mary and her brother and sister under her wing.

When Henry died in 1547, Edward became king at only nine years of age. Edward was a devout Protestant, but Mary remained faithful to her Catholic faith, which caused more distance between the siblings. Edward would only reign as king for six years, and after his death in 1553, half of England remained Catholic and wanted a Catholic queen.

When Mary took the throne, she was 37 years old and time had not been kind to her. The turmoil of her childhood had taken its toll. Any beauty that she had as a young girl had faded, and she was said to be short and unattractive with a bulky stature. Instead of a virtuous young woman, Mary Tudor was considered an old maid.

To be an effective Catholic queen, she needed a Catholic husband. In July 1554, she married Prince Philip of Spain (1527–1598), her second cousin. While Mary was quite smitten with her new husband, he did not share the same affection for her, noting that she was 'not arousing to the pleasures of the flesh'.

It is at this point in Mary's life that I must stop and consider the possibility that she may have inherited some of the mental instability that plagued her aunt, Juana the Mad. By the time Mary took the throne, she was intent on bringing England back to Catholicism and producing a male heir. But at 37, time was not on her side. She had several leaders of the Protestant Church, including those involved in her parents' divorce, executed. She declared her parents' marriage once again valid, even though they were both dead. She also reinstated the Heresy Laws, under which she burned almost 300 Protestants at the stake. It was these atrocities that earned her the title 'Bloody Mary'.

Being burned at the stake was considered one of the most gruesome deaths one could endure, and if you were lucky, you would die from inhaling carbon monoxide before burning to death. The people of England did not look upon their queen favourably for her choice of revenge on Protestants. The burnings were so unpopular that even Mary's husband and his advisers condemned them.

Things didn't get any easier for Mary Tudor. Her desperation to produce an heir to the Tudor throne almost mimicked that of her father. However, the responsibility to deliver a healthy child fell solely on Mary, and she didn't have the luxury of changing spouses in the hope of a better outcome.

It is at this time in her life that I must question her mental status again, as I compare it to that of her mother's sister. Like Juana, Mary fully devoted herself to her husband and was intent on being a dutiful wife. It is believed that Philip was faithful to Mary, but it was clear that he didn't feel the same way regarding the marriage bed. He did not find Mary attractive and was bothered by the fact that she was eleven years older than him.

Mary's health had never been very good, and her menstrual cycle only added to her malaise. She was 15 years old at the onset of her cycle, and the situation with her father and Anne Boleyn had already caused what doctors considered some form of hysteria. For years, Mary suffered from painful periods, debilitating migraines, and mood swings. Mary stated she often felt deep times of depression throughout her life. While it's impossible to be sure about what caused her menstrual troubles, endometriosis and ovarian cysts should be considered, and likely contributed to her infertility.

In the autumn of 1554, Queen Mary's menstrual cycles stopped, and she found herself plagued with nausea. She had also started to gain weight. This led her doctors to the conclusion that she must be pregnant. Mary would be required to enter her confinement roughly six weeks before the expected birth, which was believed to be in May. Mary's doctors were secretly nervous regarding the birth of her child, as they didn't see a positive outcome. Mary was 38 years old, and her mental state was not stable. Her appetite had also diminished considerably, and her doctors feared for the child's nutrition.

In late April 1555, rumours of a healthy son began to surface, and people throughout England began to celebrate. In May, however, Francisco de Eraso, a secretary to Charles V, received note that the queen's deliverance of a son was false news. Mary's abdomen had continued to swell as she awaited the birth of an heir, but the spring of 1555 came and went without any signs of the queen going into labour.

By July, there was still no sign of a new baby, but the queen simply stated that her timing must have been off, and the child would arrive soon. She also believed that God may have been punishing her and delivered a statement that until all the Protestants were punished,

God would not allow her child to be born. This lunacy began another round of brutal executions.

By the end of the summer, Mary's abdomen started to decrease in size. While everyone else seemed to figure out there would be no baby, Mary still had hope. Perhaps her delusions were made worse by the fact that Philip had left England to join his army, which was fighting the French. This left Mary utterly heartbroken.

On 11 August 1555, Queen Mary finally emerged from her confinement. She was silent, incredibly thin, and utterly humiliated. No word of the pregnancy would ever be mentioned again.

Since her youth, Mary had suffered from retention of her menstrual fluids, which caused her belly to swell, giving the appearance of a pregnancy. During the spring of 1555, Mary's breasts also began to enlarge, which would have added to the impression that she was pregnant. Mary was suffering from what would have been called a phantom pregnancy, but considering her symptoms, it's quite possible that she had some form of endometriosis or ovarian cancer. Her pelvic pain, fatigue, abdominal swelling, and irregular menstrual cycles are all symptoms of ovarian cancer.

Philip returned in 1557 and Mary soon claimed she was pregnant once again. But no baby was born, and her health was rapidly declining. She continued suffering from stomach pain, fatigue, and migraines, and in November of 1558, Mary died at the age of 42.

Margaret Tudor Sister to the King

If we look at Mary's father's side of the family, we can also see a connection to her aunt, Princess Margaret Tudor (1498–1541). Not so much in the scope of mental illness, but physical illness, specifically obstetrical and gynaecological. Margaret was born in 1489 to Henry VII and Elizabeth of York. She spent much of her childhood in the nursery at the palace of Eltham with her brother and sister, and her education most likely included learning French and studying music.

In 1503, at the age of 14, she married her third cousin James of Scotland (1473–1513), who was sixteen years older but did not give birth to their first child until February 1507. Margaret's grandmother and namesake, Margaret Beaufort, had been married at the age of 12 and gave birth to her son, Henry Tudor, at age 13. It was a traumatic birth that rendered her unable to have any future children. Margaret insisted that her granddaughter be spared the agony she had to endure, making sure some years had passed before she became pregnant. She understood that because she carried the same very thin and small frame as her grandmother, birthing children at such a young age would have been disastrous and cruel.

Sadly, one year later, her first child, would die. During her son's first and only year of life, Margaret was in a 'desperate state of health' and 'sore vexed with sickness that year'.[1] So much so, that her husband made a pilgrimage to the shrine of Ninian at Whithorn to pray for her.

Throughout the ten years of their marriage, Margaret Tudor and James would have six children, yet only one would survive childhood. A pattern of serious illness after each pregnancy plagued Margaret as she was 'grievously ill during each confinement'. She became pregnant shortly after the death of her first son and delivered a baby girl in July of 1508, who died shortly after the birth. During her marriage to James IV, she gave birth to three more children who would not live past the age of two. Her only surviving child was born in 1512 and would go on to reign as James V (1512–1542).

James IV was killed in the Battle of Flodden, and Margaret would marry twice more in her life, with each marriage producing one child, one of which also died in infancy. Her surviving daughter, Margaret Douglas (1517–1578), was born in 1517 and again, Margaret was confined to her bed for weeks after the delivery. She suffered from severe pain in her right leg, a poor appetite and developed both fevers and rashes. Margaret Tudor died on 18 October 1541, possibly of a stroke.

Margaret's son, James V, seemed to exhibit signs of mental strain, proving the possibility that he may have inherited some form of mental illness through his distant family member, Catherine of Valois. James became king when he was just 17 months old and would reign with his mother as regent until he was old enough to rule. As a young king, James was said to be handsome, charming, and skilled in riding and combat.

His mental health soon fell under duress as he feared Scottish nobles would rise against him. During the day, he was said to be: 'so retired, sullen and melancholy that everything displeased him, and he became even unsupportable to himself'. In the evenings, the king saw: 'dark shadows of displeasure, which gave terrible affright in his sleep.'[2]

Perhaps James was having nightmares about the future of Scotland.

In 1542, the king again became incapacitated and unable to lead his troops into northern England. He decided to go to Lochmaben Castle and await the outcome of the battle with the English. In a letter penned to his wife, he wrote: 'I have been ill these three days last, as I never was in my life.'[3]

On 25 November 1542, Henry VIII and his English troops defeated the Scots at Solway Moss. When King James received word on this defeat, he became very distraught and wandered aimlessly back to Edinburgh, feeling ill and demoralised. After retiring to Hallyards in Fife, he declared that in 15 days, he would be dead:

'You will be masterless and the realm without a King'[4]

The queen was in her last month of pregnancy and gave birth to a daughter. The news was brought to the king, but it did nothing to restore his melancholy. He stayed incapacitated in his bed and died on 14 December. He was only 30 years old.

It is generally believed that King James V died from severe melancholy and a broken heart. After the defeat of his army, he went into a deep depression. His defences were in disarray, and he feared the English would rule Scotland. His degree of depression makes us wonder whether it was something inherent, rather than just a situational case of melancholy. His trance-like state with repeated phrases and his wandering from town to town do seem suggestive of severe depression which perhaps came to a head with the victory of the English. The throne of Scotland was left to his daughter, Mary (Stuart) Queen of Scots, who was just six days old when she was declared queen.

Mary Stuart Queen of Scots

Mary Stuart, like her father, seemed to suffer from an 'incurable malady' for most of her life. Mary was born prematurely and was said to be a sickly child. Scotland would be ruled by regents until Mary was of age to reign. At age 5, Mary was sent to live in France in political asylum, where she would spend the next thirteen years. At age 16, she was wed to Francis the Dauphin of France, and the two would soon be crowned king and queen of France.

In the neighbouring country of England, Henry VIII's Protestant daughter, Elizabeth, inherited the crown upon the death of her sister Mary, and became Queen of England in January 1559. In the eyes of many English Catholics, however, Mary Stuart had a right to the throne, as she was the oldest legitimate descendant of Henry VII through her grandmother, Margaret Tudor. Many in England still questioned Elizabeth's legitimacy as her mother, Anne Boleyn, was often referred to as 'The Great Whore'. In France, King Henri II even went as far as to publicly proclaim his son and new daughter-in-law, king and queen of England and France. Mary's claim to the English throne would prove to be a major problem between herself and Elizabeth.

Mary's teenage years were filled with several bouts of illness that would follow her for the rest of her life. Along with tremendous stomach pains, Mary was said to be pale in colour and short of breath. A particular attack in 1563 lasted a month, and Mary suffered not only pain in her stomach, but profound periods of depression and weeping followed by sudden bursts of joy. In December of 1560, Francis died after complications from an ear infection, leaving Mary a widow; we can question whether her depressive state was a result of this event.

In 1565, Mary married English nobleman Henry Stuart, Lord Darnley, and in June of 1566, she gave birth to the future James VI of Scotland and James I of England. Shortly after the birth of her son, the queen of Scots became seriously ill, with abdominal pain, vomiting, insomnia, convulsions, and a loss of her senses. She slipped into a coma, where she lay unconscious for several days before waking. Mary feared for her life and asked for prayers before she slipped into another coma. Her doctors also feared for her life and noted that her legs 'became cold and rigid as if she had died'. Her arms and legs were massaged by her physicians, and she was then bound tightly and given sips of wine. She was given a purge, and she vomited blood but slowly recovered.

The reasons for this attack are unknown. Some historians say it may have been a form of autumnal malaria, or perhaps it was a result of the quarrelsome relationship she had with her new husband. Their marriage would not last; Lord Darnley was killed in 1567 after an explosion. As a result of her husband's death, Mary suffered terrible pains in her side, and it took her almost a month to recover. Though their marriage was turbulent, it is possible that this event only added to the stress Mary would face later in life.

Shortly after Darnley's death, the queen married James Hepburn, 4th Earl of Bothwell. It is speculated that he may have been to blame for Darnley's death, as it was believed he was having relations with Mary. After a miscarriage the following year, Mary again suffered from bouts of stomach pain and fainting. The year following, she continued to suffer with weak legs and pain in her arms in a series of attacks that came without warning. The queen wrote of her attacks in 1570, describing them in great detail to her physician. She spoke of:

> continual distillation from her head into her stomach, where of hath grown such debility and weakness in that part that she hath no desire to eat meat and is troubled with

incessant provocation to vomit. There is great pain in her left side, under the short ribs. Whether it be inflammation of the stomach, the spleen, the womb, or all of those three parts together.[5]

The queen could not sleep for days on end and was so weak she was unable to stand. She was plagued by what her doctors described as 'vehement fits of the brain'.[6]

Mary would fall ill several more times, but it is not without mentioning her turbulent life. Her marriage to Lord Bothwell was not without controversy, as many Catholics saw the marriage as illegitimate since Lord Bothwell was divorced. After an uprising against the couple in 1567, Mary was imprisoned in Loch Leven Castle before fleeing south and seeking protection from Queen Elizabeth I of England (1533–1603). However, Elizabeth only saw Mary as a threat to her throne, holding her captive for almost twenty years. She was found guilty of plotting Elizabeth's assassination and was condemned to beheading in 1587.

Many accused Mary of faking her illnesses for political gain. While she exhibited many physical symptoms, we must consider that there lies the possibility that she also suffered some sort of depression like her father, or at the least, a heightened level of anxiety, which may or may not have been inherited.

If we push ahead through several generations, we see again that defective genes continue to weave their way through European Royalty.

Chapter Seven

House of Hanover and Mad King George

England had been under Stuart rule for eleven years which ended with the Act of Settlement in 1701. Queen Anne (1665–1714), who was Queen of England, Scotland and Ireland, died in 1714. The Act of Settlement was designed so that only a Protestant could succeed to the throne of Great Britain.

Anne's story of child-rearing is a long and tumultuous one. In all, she would have seventeen pregnancies, with only five being live births, and none of her children would survive to adulthood to claim the throne of England.

Her cousin, George Ludwig (1660–1727), was the closest living Protestant relative and would inherit the crown. However, he would do so as a monarch that had no urge to learn English and cared little about adopting Great Britain as his new land.

Born in the city of Hanover, in the Duchy of Brunswick-Luneburg, on 28 May 1660, George Ludwig, was the only heir to his father's German Territories. He was described by his mother as a sensible and attentive child growing up with good health. And as a man and king, George I was physically active and enjoyed frequent hunting trips and long walks in the country.

In 1682, George would marry his first cousin, Sophia Dorothea of Celle (1666–1726), though their marriage was not without scandal. Upon being told who she was to marry, Sophia claimed, 'I will not marry a pig snout,'[1] before hurling his portrait across the room and falling to the floor in distress. And George was terribly unenthusiastic about his future bride as well.

With their marriage being quiet miserable, George much preferred his mistress, Melusine von der Schulenburg, Duchess of Kendal and Sophia had her own affair with Swedish Count, Philipp Christoph von Königsmarck (1665–1694). In 1694, the count was murdered, probably on George's orders, and his body was ruthlessly thrown into the River Leine and then butchered before it was buried beneath the floorboards of Sophia's rooms. Still, it is claimed that neither George nor Sophia had any idea where Philip's remains were.

George remained incredibly hostile to his wife, thereafter, having her sent back to Celle, where she was locked away for more than thirty years. Sophia was denied any access to the couple's two children and was kept strictly within the grounds of Ahlden House. She died in 1726 from liver failure.

But Sophia did get her revenge on her husband. While she lay suffering before her death, she penned one last letter to him. In her letter, she stated that she had cursed him for his cruelty to her. Interestingly, after receiving his wife's letter, George I died at age 67.

Throughout his life, George had a fairly blasé attitude towards medicine and assumed fate would decide in the end. Though it seemed with his wife's curse, fate was right on track. In June of 1727, the king developed severe abdominal pain, which was attributed to the fruit he had for dinner. After becoming pale and fainting, he was bled. But he eventually went into a coma and died.

While George Ludwig may have died without a long history of illness, was it his marriage to a first cousin that sparked the lengthy maladies that would eventually affect his grandson?

George Ludwig's son, George Augustus (1683–1760), would rule England upon the death of his father. As a child and young man, George II had much ill will towards his father because of how his mother had been treated. While the feeling seemed mutual, George I didn't want his son to endure a loveless marriage as he had. He gave him the opportunity to approve of his bride before any formal plans were set in place.

George spent much of his youth as a healthy man who enjoyed long walks. He seemed to share the same attitude toward sickness as his father. Lord John Hervey (1696–1743), a member of the king's privy council, noted that:

> There is a strange affection of an incapacity of being sick that ran through the whole royal family, which they carried so far that no one of them was more willing to own any other of the family ill than to acknowledge themselves to be so. I have known the king to get out of his bed, choking with a sore throat and a high fever, only to dress and have a levee, and in five minutes undress and return to his bed till the same ridiculous farce of health was to be presented the next day at the same hour.[2]

In 1705, George II met his prospective bride, Caroline of Ansbach (1683–1737), and was quite taken by her. They were married later that year in Hanover. Caroline would go on to have eight children, one dying in infancy. Prince Fredrick Ludwig (1707–1751), was heir apparent to the English throne, but died at the age of 44.

While the king enjoyed good health for most of his life, there were a few events that stood out. In October 1735, after returning from a visit to Hanover, he was feverish and suffering from painful piles, which developed after sitting for long hours in his coach. In 1737, after another visit to Hanover, George was again plagued by piles and a sore throat, fever, and cough. While attempts were made to relieve his suffering, the king felt that his physicians were: 'troublesome, inquisitive pygmies who were always plaguing him with asking impertinent, silly questions about his health like so many old nurses.'[3]

In late October of 1760, George II fell while using the privy and died later that day at the age of 77. His autopsy revealed that there had been an acute dissection of the aorta, which may have been from straining to have a bowel movement. Large amounts of pooled blood were found around his heart, which would have decreased his blood flow, eventually causing the king to lose consciousness before falling from the toilet.

George II may not stand out as one of the remembered kings of England. However, his grandson, George III (1738–1820), would go down in history as the 'Mad King'. But first, we must look at the health of two of George II's children, as it relates to genetic traits that may have been passed down.

Frederick Lewis (1707–1751), the heir presumptive, was a sickly child who was regularly purged by court physicians. By the age of 2, he had developed weak, crooked legs and a pigeon chest. Doctors suspected rickets, and Frederick was instructed to spend more time in the sun. He eventually recovered but seemed a physically weak young man. He was given a whalebone corset to help him stand upright when at court, giving off a false sense of strength. Frederick suffered from fevers and general pain and was fed ass's milk and bled to strengthen his system.

In 1736, Frederick married Princess Augusta of Saxe-Coburg (1719–1722) and two years later, their son, George Frederick was born. He was the first Hanoverian heir to the throne who was born in England.

In the winter of 1751, Frederick Lewis died, aged 44. He developed a severe cough with chest pain and fever before passing away. His post-mortem revealed that he had most likely suffered from pneumonia and died as a result of an abscess in his chest.

Frederick's younger sister, Caroline (1713–1757), would also die at the age of 44. Though she was thought of as something of a hypochondriac, she was reported to have suffered from intermittent but severe rheumatic pain that came and went. It is also believed that Caroline may have endured the same ailment as her brother.

When George Frederick was born on 4 June 1738 at St James Square, he was two months premature but was well cared for by his wet nurse, Mary Smith, and developed into a healthy, plump child. His health was good, and he was well-educated in topics that would prove useful to any prospective monarch. He learned music, language, agriculture among other subjects.

By the age of 8, he could read and write both German and English, and by 11, he was made Knight of the Garter by his grandfather. His schooldays were long and filled with geometry, Latin, writing, arithmetic and French. His mother would often sit and study more with him after dinner. Academically, he never excelled as his tutors had hoped. George was shy as a young man, but he was kind. He was also insecure about his future.

After the death of his father in 1751 and his grandfather in 1760, George Frederick ascended the throne of Great Britain as George III. He soon married Princess Sophia Charlotte of Mecklenburg-Strelitz (1744–1818) in 1761. After a rough labour, the couple welcomed their first child into the world in August 1762; in August of 1763, they welcomed their second child and, two years later, their third. The couple would go on to have fifteen children, thirteen of which would survive into adulthood.

George and Sophia's early marriage was cordial, and George was always kind to Sophia. He even discarded his wig and let his beard grow as she found it attractive. The king ensured his wife was served plenty of German meals so she would feel more at home. However, George himself had no taste for rich foods and preferred smaller meals like soups and fruits. The couple both enjoyed music, especially Johann Christian Bach. In 1764, the king welcomed eight-year-old Wolfgang Mozart to play in his court, and he was utterly delighted with him.

The king was not terribly fond of large gatherings and was often in bed by 11 pm after saying his prayers. George was a religious man who attended the Anglican Church faithfully. He also strove to be a kind monarch who paid attention to public affairs. He deemed to root out corruption and stopped the spending of the public's money on frivolous things. As a king, he was popular with his subjects and was often greeted by large crowds whenever he passed through the streets of London.

Although the king was an attentive father throughout his reign, as well as striving to be a good husband and monarch, he would spend much of his reign plagued with illness.

The king enjoyed good health and remained physically active until, in 1762 at the age of 22, he became ill with what was described as a 'feverish cold'. A violent cough, along with severe tightness in his chest developed; he also had a fast pulse and suffered with constipation. Doctors were sure he had consumption and prescribed him laxatives and ass's milk. He was also bled over half-a-dozen times, but it would be weeks before he felt well enough to return to his normal activities.

In 1763, problems with the king's administration began to develop, and he often expressed his agitation to the queen. He complained about his ministers being insolent and lacking duty, and he had a generally gloomy attitude about him.

In 1765, an attack similar to the one of 1762 occurred. Again, the king developed a cough and fever, along with tightness in his chest and a hoarse voice. His pulse raced, and he found he could only sleep a few hours each night. He was bled and cupped by doctors and did not feel well again until the summer of that same year. During this time, the king feared for his own life and instructed his ministers to propose a bill that would appoint a regent to rule if he should die before his heir reached legal age.

It would be over twenty years before the king would fall ill again. During those years, he continued to serve his country through the American War of Independence. He was enraged by the British Patriots who supported the Americans, Thomas Payne and Benjamin Franklin being two of the most famous. In the summer of 1788, George III began complaining of severe abdominal pain and constipation, along with muscle weakness and stiffness in the legs. His condition continued to deteriorate as he suffered a racing pulse, insomnia, and incessant talking. He took to his bed, and following an examination by his doctors, he was diagnosed with gout as they claimed his bile was not flowing correctly.

Feeling dissatisfied with the treatment of his physicians, he refused any further medicines and decided to go to Cheltenham Spa in the Cotswolds for a course in the waters. He drank three glasses of water a day and reported that he felt a bit better as the water acted as a purge. Doctors there: 'removed bile in a very gentle manner. They strengthened the stomach and are a gentle brace to the constitution.'[4]

While at Cheltenham, he made several trips to an Abbey in Tewksbury, where he was seen wandering around eccentrically, walking into the homes of random strangers to simply say hello.

Upon returning to Windsor in August of that year, the king's severe stomach pains returned, along with laboured breathing and leg cramps. He developed a rash on his arm, along with a racing pulse, insomnia, and an inability to concentrate on his work. His physician, George Baker (1722–1809), felt that the king's illness may have been from walking outside in wet stockings, but all his physicians generally agreed that gout was the most likely culprit.

His condition worsened to the point he would ramble on for hours without pause, causing foam to develop at the corner of his mouth. He developed a horse voice and became agitated. The king would repeat himself over and over again, sometimes speaking over 400 words without taking a breath, with a vocabulary that became more creative and complex. His physician noted that he continued to suffer acute pain in his stomach, which spread to his back and sides, making it difficult to breathe. Baker also noted that the king's urine was a brownish colour. His memory continued to deteriorate, and he became delirious at times and was unable to focus on government business long enough to pen a letter. After showing daughter, Princess Elizabeth (1770–1840), a rash that had developed on his arm, she said it was very red and 'in great weals as if it had been scourged with cords'.[5]

Baker was still convinced the king's ailments were because he had walked on the grass too long and his socks were wet. He also blamed the king's illness on the four pears he had consumed for dinner prior to getting sick. One October morning, Baker was called after the king

suffered from a painful 'spasmodic bilious attack'. He complained
of severe belly and side pain and was given laudanum after a large
bowel movement. He worsened with a fever and swollen feet, and
his urine took on a brownish hue. The king was weak, contributing to
his inability to write letters to conduct affairs. At the end of October,
the king went into a rage and yelled at Baker about the medications
he had been given.

Baker recorded, 'the look in his eyes, the tone of his voice, every
gesture and his whole deportment represented a person in a most
furious passion of anger. One medicine was too powerful, and another
only teased him without effect.'[6]

On 24 October the king demanded to appear at the levee to let
people know he was quite well, and there was no case for alarm. But
upon doing so, he looked so dishevelled that the Lord Chancellor
had to ask him to adjust his outfit as his legs were wrapped in
flannel, his speech was slurred, and he appeared hurried and agitated.
He rambled on with muddled thought and didn't seem to have any
understanding that his appearance was disastrous. In a letter penned
by Fanny Burney, she states:

> He assures everybody of his health. He was all benevolence
> and goodness, even to the degree that made it touching to
> hear him speak. Yet, he spoke in a manner so uncommon
> that a high fever alone could not account for it. A rapidity,
> a hoarseness of voice, a volubility, an earnestness, a
> vehemence rather. It startled me inexpressibly.[7]

The queen grew increasingly uneasy about her husband's health,
especially when she heard him conversing with Mrs Fanny Burney,
her Keeper of the Wardrobe (1752–1840). The king talked to
Mrs Burney often, telling her about his health woes. He told her how
he hardly slept and asked her to remind the queen not to talk to him
before bed. The queen was not only uneasy but becoming scared of
her husband, although he was quite dependent on her. Of the queen,

he said: 'The queen is my physician, and no man need have better, and no man can have a better.'[8]

Mrs Burney had her own observations about how the king would sweat profusely, drench his clothes, seemed very irritated and was easily offended. However, at other times, she observed him to be in good humour and good spirits as he walked around singing.

Sophia was worried by the king's 'great hurry and spirits and incessant loquacity'[9], and called for Dr Baker. When Baker arrived, the king acted as if he was listening to a concert but there was no music as the symphony was all in his head. He was talking and moving about from room to room and from one subject to another as he waved his arms as if directing a full orchestra. The king told his physician that there was pain and weakness in his knee; he kept rising and then sitting down repeatedly and confessed that he was sure he was going deaf. The king seemed to understand that he may be losing his mind because once he began talking, he could not stop. His attendants tried to calm him by reading to him, but he kept talking for what seemed like hours.

His rambles would continue for days at a time and at one point, he suddenly burst into tears on the Duke of York's (1763–1827) shoulder and said, 'I wish to God I may die, for I am gone to be mad.'[10]

The king's children were entirely distraught by his condition; during a dinner with the queen and his children he grew very irritated, rose from the table, grabbed The Duke of York by the collar and threw him against the wall. Dr Baker stated that after this outburst, it appeared the king was now: 'under an entire alienation of the mind and much more agitated than he had ever been. The pulse was so very quick, 120 the next morning but fewer than 100 after being bled.'[11]

The queen stated: 'his eyes were like black currant jelly, the veins in his face were swollen, and the sound of his voice dreadful. He spoke until he was exhausted, and the moment he recovered his breath, he began again, while foam ran from his mouth.'[12]

That night the king stood over her bed and stared at her. She awoke and moved to another room, and the king was persuaded to return to his rooms, but people were afraid to approach him. Later that next day, Dr Baker said the king was still very agitated, sweating and complaining of burning as he continued to ramble on for hours. Baker soon became very overwhelmed with treating the king.

The king's son, the Prince of Wales (1762–1830), called upon his own doctor, Richard Warren (1731–1797), to examine his father. However, the queen was not in favour of Dr Warren, and so the king ordered him out of his rooms, shoving him while foaming at the mouth. Warren reported that the king's mind had gone deranged as he witnessed him talk until he was exhausted. The king began hallucinating and talking with people who were long dead. He suffered convulsions and went into a coma. Warren, along with the king's doctors, agreed that he could not perform his duties as king and did not know if there was hope for recovery. They were unsure if his ailment was in the brain alone or another part of his body.

The treatments prescribed to the king consisted of his head being shaved and then blistered, to draw the poison from his brain. His legs were also blistered with plasters of cantharides and mustard, which was believed to draw the humours in the opposite direction. He was given purges and enemas, leeches were put on his forehead, he was given a sedative, and his room was kept terribly cold with no fire lit.

On the king's calmer days, he was able to take a warm bath, and he would allow his doctors to shave his head, but there was still no improvement. He had insomnia and convulsions that were so bad his pages had to hold him in fear that he would injure himself. George sometimes treated his pages horribly, slapping them in the face, kicking them, and pulling their hair. And then it was as if a wave of compassion overcame him, and he would feel terribly bad and beg their forgiveness.

As the king grew thin and fragile, there was talk of the Prince of Wales becoming regent, and a bill was finally introduced to appoint him as so.

On 6 November, the king was given a dose of James's Powder for the reduction of his fever, and this caused him to have a huge bowel movement before he fell asleep. Upon waking from this sleep, the king raved like a lunatic and howled like a dog. His doctors were convinced that he was becoming totally mad, and Dr Warren said it was direct lunacy and that he may never recover. However, others felt that he would make a recovery, and these two differing opinions caused the newspapers to run stories that caused utter confusion for many. The people of London began to wonder if the king's doctors were nothing more than a bunch of quacks. His physicians felt that a move from Windsor to Kew would be appropriate, where he could walk in the gardens in peace.

The queen was becoming more distraught and disgusted by her husband's behaviour and endless talking. He would cry in front of her and tell her she was ignoring him and breaking his heart. She was getting almost no sleep at night. The queen appeared as though she might also suffer a nervous breakdown herself at times and was often found to be sitting with her head in her hands, crying.

When the king was informed that his doctors wanted to move him to Kew, he said he would only go if the queen were going to be there. However, when Dr Warren tried to convince him of that, the king assaulted him, and he had to be removed from Windsor by force. Upon discovering that the queen really wasn't going to be at Kew, the king again threw a temper tantrum and assaulted his men. That night he refused to sleep and instead began hopping around his rooms. The king had to be tied to his bed while he begged his attendants to end his life. He also had burst of childlike behaviour where he would ask his pages to wheel him around his room.

The king's doctors examined an oath from the Privy Council that addressed the king's situation. The council agreed that the king was not capable of tending to his affairs. Newspapers continued to print stories about the king's health. Another doctor was called to see the king that December. Dr Francis Willis (1718–1807), who was not only a physician but an Anglican priest, successfully treated mentally ill patients. The 70-year-old clergyman was recommended by the Lord Chancellor, but it was said that he practised without a license, even though he had a degree from Oxford University. Dr Willis had successfully treated mentally ill patients at a hospital in Lincoln, and he opened his own asylum at Gretford. While Dr Willis was effective, the other physicians who treated the king questioned his work. He was not a member of the Royal College and had something of a tarnished reputation due to his practising without a license. His Majesty was not overly impressed with Dr Willis either and assured him he was much better and needed no help.

However, despite the king's opinion, members of the royal household did like Dr Willis. They believed he was open and honest and should be given much credit for his work treating the mentally ill. While his patients stayed at Gretford, they were expected to pay a fee for their care. The patients were treated well, ate meals together, and were also encouraged to socialise with one another.

Dr Willis had some treatments that we may question today but were considered acceptable and appropriate at the time. He favoured restraints, including the straightjacket, which would be used on the king when he was unruly. Willis used the straightjacket as a threat when the king refused to cooperate in simple tasks such as eating, or when he refused to leave his bed. Willis also used a special type of chair to ensure the king's compliance, where he would have the king strapped to the chair with a cloth stuffed in his mouth; the king would then be verbally reprimanded. He was also served a bland diet that could only be consumed with a spoon as it was feared he might try to harm himself. There were even times when the king would ask for the straightjacket so he could be still enough to sleep.

Willis's notes included a document of how the king's 'tongue was whitish, pulse 108, under constraint most of the day'.[13]

George's treatments continued, where he was blistered and given calomel, camphor, digitalis, and tartarised antimony, which made him so sick that he often fell to his knees praying for death.

During his more subdued times, the king did agree that Dr Willis calmed him – as much as he hated to admit it. It was noticed that when agitated, the king would relax once Dr Willis came into the room. He let the king shave himself under his supervision, which had not been done previously. He was also allowed to cut his toenails and spend time with his dog, Flora, who brought him much joy.

While the king's separation from his wife was hard on him, over the next two months, he was able to visit with his family and walk the grounds with them. They spoke of his horses and the current affairs of the English army, and doctors agreed that he was coherent again. The Lord Chancellor also decided that it would be unnecessary to proceed further with the Regency Bill, and he could begin official business again. Public support for the king during this time was shown with celebration concerts and balls. In April of 1789, the king rode into London and was moved by his citizens singing, 'God Save the king.'

Despite his visits with family, the king would sometimes become so agitated that he would be put in his straightjacket at 4 pm and not let out until the following morning; he seemed to go through periods where he was lucid and coherent, and then confused and incoherent again.

The king's relationship with the queen was one with many ups and downs due to his mental illness. He would often cry, stating that he missed his wife, but he would also tell her directly that he was not fond of her that day. From 1788–93, the king refused to allow the queen into his bed without explanation. In 1789, the queen had a plump and delicious bunch of grapes sent to the king, who sent them back without a word. The king also asked for the queen's dog, Badine, to keep him company, stating that he favoured the dog over her. He then stated that the queen had a foul temper, and all the children feared her.

By the end of December of 1789, the queen was distraught over her husband, exhausted and lacking in appetite. She would sit alone and cry, not only for her husband's behaviour but for her son as well. The Prince of Wales seemed irritated by his mother's distress, and he had a cold demeanour with her and didn't pay her much attention.

George's doctors still seemed to have conflicting opinions about his recovery. Dr Willis felt strongly that the king was improving, while other's felt he was acting very disturbed and the straightjacket should be used again. It seemed as if the king's doctors couldn't agree on something as simple as his heart rate. By the middle of January the following year, Dr Baker said the king had relapsed into a 'state of total alienation'[14], despite short periods of lucidity.

At one point, the queen accompanied him on what she envisioned as a quiet ride through Richmond Park, but the king suddenly became violent and needed to be restrained. He was irritable for days after this event and was given an enema that, as usual, made him so sick that he prayed for death. After a period of calmness, the king was brought to a pagoda in the Kew Gardens when he tried to run off. He climbed to the top of the pagoda and, after being brought down, threw himself on the ground, where he lay for over 45 minutes. He was once again restrained and brought back inside.

Still, doctors argued that the king's rages were becoming less common and pointed out that he had lovingly fed the queen's dog before putting a little blue bow around his neck. There was also the time that the queen spent over an hour in the king's rooms before they both emerged, looking quite content. The night before the queen's birthday, the king appeared calm and pleasant; but by the end of the day, he was throwing chairs at the housekeepers, but later that evening, he was calm again and had a nice dinner with the queen and three of their sons.

At one point during one of the queen's visits, she was accompanied by Mrs Burney, who found herself quite startled when the king suddenly rushed towards her, yelling for her to stop. Because the queen instructed there was to be no contact with the king, she turned away from him. She said: 'There was something of wildness in his eyes. Think, however, of my surprise to feel him put both his hands around my two shoulders and kiss my cheek.'[15]

The king then went on to tell Mrs Burney that he was doing quite well and had never felt better, before divulging a story about how he disliked all his pages.

Towards the end of 1800, the king again fell into a period of calmness where he was allowed to shave himself and would visit his farm animals and play his flute. The king was sure he no longer needed doctors and so dismissed them. He appeared to have fully recovered and spent time with the queen, his children, and his animals. He personally visited a lunatic asylum in Richmond to enquire about the treatments being used. He declared that the straightjacket was the best thing that had happened to him.

By the end of February that year, the king's doctors finally agreed that he was 'free from complaint', and the city of London rejoiced in his recovery with lavish balls and parties.

George III's recovery did not last long because, in February 1801, he suffered again from the same afflictions after catching a chill. He was plagued with stomach pain, constipation, brown urine, a racing pulse, and a hoarse voice. He also talked incessantly. However, this time he was able to voice his concerns to the queen as well as Dr Willis. 'I am much more weaker than I was, and I pray to God all night that I might die or that He would spare my reason.'[16]

George became lethargic and delirious and fell into a coma, where he appeared to worsen dramatically. The following is an excerpt from the diary of Dr Willis from 1 March 1801:

> His Majesty's fever increased in the afternoon, and his night having been very restless and unquiet. At the recommendation of Dr Reynolds, His Majesty's feet were put into hot water and vinegar for half an hour. Soon after this, His Majesty put on such an appearance of being exhausted that his life was despaired of – his pulse too had rapidly increased.[17]

That same evening, several of the king's doctors offered their opinions on his health and continued treatment.

> They gave him a strong dose of bark, containing quinine, which had the effect of composing him and putting him to sleep for an hour and a half. Before, he had been in a very

100

restless and unquiet state. He walked with a slower pulse and in every respect appearing better…his medicines of today since 2 o'clock were chiefly composed of musk and bark-his nourishment jellies and wine.[18]

The components used to rid the king's body of toxins were antimony-based James powders, purgatives, arsenicals, and tartar emetics. Unknown at the time, the doctors were giving the king an alarmingly high rate of arsenic, most likely poisoning him, and causing encephalopathy.

Despite this, Dr Willis claimed the king did recover because, on 5 March, he was again sitting up and eating. He met with the queen and his children and said he felt much better.

> He laid aside all false pretences, all petty vexations, all unnecessary restraints; no violence needed to be apprehended and that no suspicion should be shown. The good effects of the altered treatment speedily appeared. As yet, the delusions continued unabated, but far greater calmness and composure, as also better health, were attained.[19]

The king would remain in recovery as he slept poorly, felt tired and weak, his eyes were dim, and he had become so thin that his clothes hung off him. He also became furious with his doctors again and said he resented their medical treatment of him. He ordered Dr Willis out of his sight before riding off to the White House at Kew.

Upon hearing about the king's angry departure, the queen permitted the guards to go after him. When they found him and entered his room, he was informed that he would be confined again and have no access to his queen. The king stated he would sign no papers relating to government until he saw the queen.

His health was sporadic over the next few months, but by May of that year, the king was eating again and was able to visit the queen.

He was also able to discuss government affairs and once again perform his official duties. Still, he found himself very tired most mornings and struggled to get out of bed. He was permitted to recover further at Weymouth with the queen by his side. On their way there, they were caught in a sudden downpour. The king refused to wear a jacket and ate his dinner that evening in soaking-wet clothes. Several days later, he assured everyone that he had been sleeping wonderfully at Weymouth and was giving up all medical treatment.

By the fall of that year, he seemed greatly improved, and when war with France broke out, he stated that he would be at the front lines with his troops to fend off enemy forces.

Sadly, in January of 1804, the king developed a respiratory infection and was again plagued by stomach pain, weakness of the limbs, agitation, and hurried speech. As his fever spiked, he rambled on for five hours straight. Charles Abbot, Speaker of the House of Commons (1757–1829), reported that his disorder had taken the 'decided character of complete mental derangement.'[20]

He soon became paralysed, and a straightjacket had to be used to control his behaviour. He once again began having strong aversions to his wife. The Duke of Kent (1767–1820) reported that there was:

> an astonishing change for the worse as the king's manner was so much more hurried, his conversation so infinitely more light and silly, his temper so much more irritable, besides a strong indication of fever on his cheek, a return of that dreadful saliva, of the strong bilious eye and of numberless symptoms that manifested themselves and proved to be a forerunner of a serious attack.[21]

Observers also reported to the prince that the king was 'so violent with his family that they all dreaded him beyond recognition'. The king soon developed a stumbling walk, became short-sighted and would stare at those he spoke to with protruding eyes and shout directly into their faces.

The queen signed a declaration that the king's cabinet, not the family, would make all future decisions about his treatment. His Prime Minister, William Pitt (1759–1806), was to see about all his care and argued that the king should be spared any mental exertion and avoid further fatigue.

As the months passed, the queen found herself under tremendous anxiety. She was thin and became ill-tempered from having to endure the king's behaviour. By the summer of 1804, she could no longer tolerate her husband's behaviour, and her daughters were also miserable. The king once again made it clear that he was quite dissatisfied with his wife.

In the summer of 1805, the king endured a new treatment where leeches were applied to his eyes for his near-sightedness to the point that they became so inflamed that he could no longer see enough to write letters. He found it hard to make out faces and could not read, even with his spectacles.

In October 1810, Britain celebrated the 50th year of George III's reign with receptions, formal balls, fireworks, and concerts. The year prior, the French were defeated at Talavera, and the king's popularity had soared. He was seen as an honest and dependable king. During the celebration of his jubilee, the king was more popular than ever.

But at the same time, the king's daughter, Princess Amelia (1783–1810), was dying of consumption, and he was heartbroken. It was incredibly hard to witness his daughter's agony from the treatment used to drain the fluid from her lungs. Perhaps it was the sickness of his child that brought on yet another attack. The king caught a cold, and the by now familiar symptoms of abdominal pain, rapid pulse and agitation were back. The king became confused and was certain his sons had fled England because the country was being flooded. He became easily distracted and unbalanced, shouting aimlessly as he rode his horse, crying out at the thought of his daughter passing away.

One of Amelia's nurses said: 'the scenes of distress and crying every day during the hours the king used to be with his daughter were melancholy beyond description'.[22]

Sadly, Princess Amelia's health deteriorated, and she developed a bacterial infection along with the consumption. She passed on 2 November 1810, and the king was devastated. He fell into a deep depression, and by mid-December it was feared that he, too, may die. While the king had delusions that his daughter was still alive, the Prince of Wales was sworn in as regent on 6 February 1811.

Over the next several months, the king faded in and out of coherence; there was a calm period in May, but he needed the straight jacket again by late October. He soon seemed to retreat into a fantasy world where he imagined the dead were once again living. The queen did her best to comfort her husband, but it seemed he had forgotten who she was, and her last visit with him was in June of 1812.

The queen's relationship with her children deteriorated, and she became more withdrawn as she spent her days alone, tending to her garden. Queen Sophia died in 1818, alone and full of sadness; the king was completely oblivious to his wife's death.

As the months passed by, the king took to wandering around, with a stooped-over posture like an entity, with his beard long. He was annoyed by almost everyone and continued to have delusions that God was bringing a flood to England. He went from laughter to tears repeatedly, and there were times when he believed he was dead. He walked aimlessly through his palace in his flannel nightgown, talking to people who had long since been dead. He spent hours upon hours tying and untying his handkerchief and buttoning and unbuttoning his coat. After saying his prayers every night, he stuffed a handkerchief in his mouth out of fear that he may say something blasphemous. It seemed his only pleasure was eating and sitting in a dark room.

By the end of 1819, the king was on a liquid diet and was observed to speak nonsense for over fifty-eight hours straight. His doctors could not agree among themselves whether he would ever fully recover. His symptoms came and went over the next few years, and he often appeared to be in another world, hardly recognising family and friends. George III finally died peacefully in 1820 on 29 of January at the age of 81.

Throughout his life, George III repeatedly suffered from attacks that seemed to start with respiratory infections or viruses. The symptoms of abdominal pain with constipation, painful limbs, rapid pulse, hoarse voice, trouble swallowing, insomnia, delusions, welts on his arms and discoloured urine remained consistent. The changes in his urine seemed to appear during the worse parts of his illness and then resolved once he recovered.

Since the Middle Ages, doctors have understood that changes in one's urine could be linked to different diseases. Urine was often collected in a flask and brought to physicians for inspection. Without visiting the patient, doctors used to diagnose based on the colour, quantity, clarity – and sometimes taste of the urine. Because of the influence of the physician Galen, doctors believed that urine was the key to gauging the health of one's liver, where blood was believed to have been produced. Physicians believed that studying urine was the best way to determine whether the patient's humours were out of balance.

The 'urine wheel' consisted of twenty colours ranging from white, to gold, to almost black. Along with the colour, the smell and taste of a patient's urine were considered an extremely important part of diagnosis and recommended treatment. Some report that King George's urine may have been so dark brown that it appeared purple. By the seventeenth century, urine wheels had become so widely printed that all sorts of people were using them, including unlicensed medical practitioners known as 'piss prophets'. The Royal College in London forbade its members to diagnose a patient solely on their urine sample and needed to consider the bigger picture of the patient's symptoms.

King George's doctors reported on the colour of his urine on four different occasions. In October of 1788, Dr George Baker noted that the urine was brown, while in January of 1811, Dr Henry Halford reported that it was a: 'deep coloured urine which left a pale blue ring upon the glass near the upper surface'. Similar blueish urine was reported in January 1812, and in August of 1819, the king's urine was reported to be like brown, bloody water.

It's hard to say what caused the king's bluish urine. Some historians are adamant the king had porphyria, a rare but complicated disease where certain chemicals in the body build up, causing a myriad of symptoms. Wilfred Arnold, a PhD at the University of Kansas Medical Centre in Kansas City, Kansas, said that the blue colour of George's urine probably resulted from the precipitation of molecules knowns as indoles in the urine. The king's chronic constipation most likely caused any tryptophan, an essential amino acid, in his diet to be metabolised to indole by the normal bowel flora. If the indole were absorbed into his blood, it would have been secreted as a colourless material in his urine. Because chamber pots were widely used and probably not cleaned very well, the indole was probably exposed to bacteria, giving the urine its blueish colour.

Whether George III, or any of the Hanoverians, suffered from porphyria is still up for debate. In the mid–1960s, two psychiatrists by the name of Ida Macalpine and Richard Hunter published a book called *George III and the Mad Business*. The book made the case that the king suffered from attacks of porphyria, which seemed to be the consensus among other historians and laypeople. Their diagnosis of the king was based on his symptoms of blindness, muscle weakness, hoarseness, stomach pain and discoloured urine, which are all prevalent in porphyria. However, the interpretation of the king's symptoms overlooked the fact that he also suffered from an altered mental state during many of his episodes. Several recent studies have challenged the diagnosis of porphyria, strongly advocating for a diagnosis of bipolar disorder, which greatly explains the waxing and waning of the king's behaviour.

Historians have since questioned the strong propensity towards porphyria by Macalpine and Hunter and have tried to understand the reason for such a passionate diagnosis.

Macalpine trained in German universities before moving to England with her two sons. She worked as an assistant psychiatrist at St Bartholomew's Hospital, where her son Richard trained. Despite his academic aspirations, he was denied chairs in psychiatry. The mother and son team published several papers with a more organic approach to psychiatry, reflected in their work on King George III. Suggesting that the king's disorder was metabolic would support their research on a more physiological cause. The pair also deemed to remove the scarlet letter of madness from the House of Hanover, something they hoped to be greatly rewarded for.

The pair gained support from distinguished biochemists, which strengthened their hypothesis. In fact, any criticism about the idea was either ignored or viciously shot down as nonsense. The claim of porphyria became well recognised, especially in theatre and film, such as in Peter Maxwell Davies's *Portraits for a Mad King.*

Macalpine and Hunter's work also brought about a myriad of claims that several other historical figures, mostly antecedents and descendants of King George, shared the diagnosis of porphyria. These claims continue to be an ongoing study today.

As the world of psychiatry grew and the knowledge of mental illness expanded, it is understood that recurrent episodes of bipolar disorder can lead to dementia, low esteem, tarnished relationships with loved ones, and a sense of living in a type of fantasy land. Bipolar disorder is also believed to be brought on, in some cases, by a stressful event in life. If we look at George III and his overwhelming loss of children, it is certainly easy to understand how this may have been the case. As a young king and husband, he lost two very small children in less than a year and was utterly devastated by these losses.

But whether it was a bipolar disorder or some other disease, it doesn't change the fact that his doctors didn't know either, and the medical treatments administered by them most likely made things worse. Despite being the best physicians of the time, the king's doctors certainly were unaware that the repeated bleeding only caused depleted blood volume, which required the heart to beat faster and the pulse to quicken. Cupping to remove the bad humours would only allow bruising and skin damage, making it a breeding ground for bacteria. And it seems likely, in the king's case, that infection may also have triggered attacks of porphyria, if that is indeed what he had.

The consistent purging of his stomach and bowels using what was believed to be the best medications at the time most certainly only irritated his digestive system and possibly damaged it. While senna is a relatively safe, natural laxative and is still used today, it can cause intense bowel spasms, which would have made the king's agitated stomach worse. Tartar emetic only irritates the bowel wall, and calomel contains not only chloride but mercury. Aloe and taraxacum (dandelions) were both laxatives which would have also caused stomach pain.

When King George was agitated, he was given laudanum, a form of opium. While it may have had a sedating effect, opium derivatives are known to cause constipation. At the time, musk was used for its calming effects as well and was often used to control seizures. However, we know today that musk can also decrease oxygen to the tissues, suppressing their ability to recover from illness.

Modern chemical analysis of hair from the king can tell us that he had elevated levels of arsenic in his body. Not only was arsenic a favourite medication prescribed by doctors, but it was also used to freshen up hair pieces. Mercury and lead were also prevalent. Mercury was often found in medications prescribed by seventeenth- and eighteenth-century doctors, and lead was most likely found in drinking water stored in lead vats.

If the king did indeed have porphyria, symptoms of the disease would be expected to appear in not only his children but his ancestors as well. When the Prince of Wales finally became George IV in 1820, he threw an elaborate coronation, which only added to his mounting debts. By the time he was king, he was morbidly obese and addicted to laudanum.

His marriage to his cousin, Princess Caroline of Brunswick (1768–1821), was disastrous from the start as neither found interest in the another. They married in 1795 and, within a year, were separated. The prince preferred the company of his mistresses instead and fathered several illegitimate children. By the time George IV ascended the throne, he and Caroline had been separated for many years, and Caroline had left England. She returned to be crowned queen, but George refused to recognise her as such and had her name removed from the Book of Common Prayer and the liturgy of the Church of England.

The king's indulgent lifestyle had caught up with him by the late 1820s. He secluded himself away at Windsor, and on the rare occasions he did appear in public, he became the target of many jokes. He spent his last years in bed, suffering from severe bouts of breathlessness. His physical and mental health worsened as he continued to draw from public affairs. By 1828, he had lost almost all his vision due to cataracts and suffered from painful gout in his right arm. The king took laudanum for his severe bladder pains, leaving him mentally fragile for days. By the time he had surgery in 1829 to remove a cataract, he was reportedly taking over 100 drops of laudanum at a time.

According to Scottish Painter, Sir David Wilkie (1785–1841), the king was: 'wasting away frightfully day after day. He had become so obese that he looked like a great sausage stuffed into the covering.'

By 1830, his attacks of breathlessness forced him to sleep sitting up, and his doctors had to continuously drain fluid from his abdomen. But still, he continued to indulge in unhealthy foods. The Duke of Wellington remarked that the king had eaten for breakfast, 'a Pidgeon and Beef Steak Pye ... Three parts of a bottle of Mozelle, a Glass of Dry Champagne, two Glasses of Port and a Glass of Brandy', followed by a large dose of laudanum.

His physician, Sir Henry Halford (1766–1844), whose treatments included administering both opium and laudanum, said the king was: 'utterly and entirely destitute of information'.

On 26 June 1830, early in the morning at Windsor Castle, he passed a large bloody stool. He sent for his physician in fear for his life. He died in the arms of his page less than ten minutes later. The king's autopsy revealed that he suffered from a gastrointestinal bleed, and a large tumour was found on his bladder. His heart was also enlarged and was surrounded by large fatty deposits.

William Henry (1765–1837), third son of George III and brother of George IV, took the throne that same day and became Britain's last monarch of the House of Hanover. He married Princess Adelaide of Saxe-Meiningen (1792–1849), but his only surviving children were illegitimate through his mistress.

When William IV died, the throne was passed to his niece, Victoria, under British law. Williams's brother Edward (1767–1820) was crowned king of Hanover, ending the union between England and the House of Hanover.

Perhaps, if we look back on the House of Hanover, it was Queen Anne from the House of Stuart who may have contributed to the many ailments of Hanover's monarchs. Her slew of failed pregnancies may tell us something about the bloodline passed to George I. Four of her five children to survive childbirth died before the age of two, leading us to question whether there was a genetic mutation.

Is it possible that she suffered from Lupus, an autoimmune disorder where the body attacks its own tissues? Anne complained of chronic pain in her limbs and headaches, which are symptoms of this genetic disease. It's also possible she suffered from diabetes, gout, or porphyria.

Queen Anne spent much of her later life in considerable pain, confined to a wheelchair. Along with weight gain, she exhibited a melancholy that was noticeable to her courtiers. With the death of her only living heir at the age of eleven, it's not hard to have pity for Queen Anne, weather or not she was responsible for the onset of porphyria and perhaps, many of the other ailments that affected the Hanoverian crown.

But nonetheless, when the crown passed to the young and vibrant Victoria in 1838, generations to come would be plagued by a devastating blood disorder.

Chapter Eight

Queen Victoria's Haemophilia Trait

On 24 May 1819, Alexandrina Victoria was born at Kensington Palace in London. Her father, Edward, Duke of Kent, was the fourth son of the mad King George. The king, as we know, had several other sons, one of which would succeed him to the throne of England. With the clustering of sons, it was assumed that one of them would certainly provide a male heir to follow in the footsteps of George IV.

Victoria's mother was Victoire of Saxe-Coburg and Princess of Leiningen (1786–1861), a small German province. While Victoria's (or Drina's, as she would soon be called) parents hoped to conceive a son, she would be the couple's only child. In January of 1820, her father died of pneumonia, followed by her grandfather, George III.

While her uncle, Prince George Fredrick Augustus, would take the throne as George IV, Victoria lived a quiet and uneventful childhood with her German-speaking household. Victoria was taught English, as well as an education in philosophy, music, history, and foreign language. Victoria was described as a mischievous, lively child with a warm and happy heart. She was said to have a romantic streak and always carried herself with dignity.

In November of 1817, two years before Victoria was born, her cousin Princess Charlotte (1796–1817), the only daughter of George IV, suffered tremendously with a distressing labour. The marriage between Charlotte's parents was one that was filled with a great amount of distaste, so it's not hard to understand why Charlotte was the only child. Her father had no favour whatsoever with her mother and much preferred his mistresses to his wife. George paid Charlotte a minimal amount of attention during her childhood, but as part of his disdain for his wife, he kept the two separated.

While Queen Victoria will always be branded as the monarch that carried the gene of haemophilia, attention must be given to her cousin Charlotte, who seemed to endure the same poor health as their grandfather, King George III. While there was no recorded knowledge of excessive bleeding in the previous king, it seems that Charlotte shared some of the same ailments – even if women could not suffer from the effects of haemophilia.

As a child, Charlotte suffered from bouts of abdominal pain which may or may not have been connected to her coming menstruation. But much like her grandfather, she dealt with insomnia and a rapid shifting of moods such as excitement and depression. While it's perfectly reasonable to assume that all these things may have been a normal part of puberty in any teenage girl, we can't ignore the fact that Charlotte's grandfather may have passed on some type of ailment to his children and grandchildren when we look at further evidence of depression. And the horrors of a bleeding disorder that were soon to come may have been tangled in the web of genetics passed down from George III, rather than starting with Victoria.

At age 18, Princess Charlotte fell deeply in love with Leopold of Coburg (1790–1865), a member of a small German ducal family. Unlike the courtship of her mother, her blossoming relationship with Leopold was filled with genuine romance and affection. The couple married in May of 1816 when Charlotte was 21 years old. She had grown into a delightful woman with a long, elegant nose and golden-brown ringlets that fell on her shoulders. Ms Fanny Burney, who had the pleasure of seeing her while she attended to the queen, described Charlotte as 'quite beautiful', and that it 'was impossible not to be struck with her personal attraction, her youth, and splendour'.[1]

Charlotte found herself pregnant within a month of her wedding but sadly miscarried the child two months later. By early 1817, she was pregnant again. While a normal gestation for a pregnant woman is forty weeks, Charlotte didn't go into labour until she was forty-two weeks. Doctors today are always cautious past the forty-week mark as complications can arise.

During the evening of 3 November 1817, at Claremont House in Surrey, Princess Charlotte's water broke, and she complained of 'sharp, acute and distressing'[2] labour pains. Sir Richard Croft (1762–1818), obstetrician and midwife, had already settled into the household a few weeks earlier to prepare for the birth. Along with Croft, Mrs Griffiths, the same wet nurse who had cared for Victoria's father as a baby, moved in as head midwife.

Around eleven o'clock, Croft examined the princess and found she was beginning to dilate. It's important to remember that this exam would not have been carried out under sterile circumstances, with no washing of the hands. Charlotte's labour was proceeding, but not as fast as the medical team would have liked. Her labour intensified, and she began vomiting in the early morning hours. Sir Richard sent for another obstetrician, Dr Baillie (1761–1823).

At 11 am a second examination was performed, only to find out that the cervix had further dilated only slightly. By this time, Croft was considering sending for a third doctor, Dr John Simms (1749–1831). Around 9 pm that evening, Charlotte's cervix was finally fully effaced, but by this time, she had been in labour well over twenty-four hours and found she was almost too weak to push.

Aside from the exhaustion of childbirth, there is a good chance that Princess Charlotte was severely anaemic. For women of the aristocracy, the recommended diet during pregnancy included very little meat and vegetables – two crucial sources of iron. Along with having low iron, the princess was bled an alarming number of times.

The practice of bloodletting was still considered the gold standard for both men and women, and especially concerning a woman's gynaecological and obstetrical procedures. If a woman's periods were too heavy, too light, or didn't come at all, she was to be bled. Obstetricians also recommended that a woman 'be bled at least three times, in the fifth, the seventh, and the last month to avoid haemorrhage and to prevent the child from growing too large'.[3]

If a woman haemorrhaged during the delivery of her child, more blood was taken from her as a remedy.

Charlotte was weak on that second night of labour; her pains were inconsistent and both Croft and Baillie knew something was wrong. This prompted Croft to summon Dr Simms, who arrived late at the night.

The use of obstetric forceps was nothing new, having been used for over 100 years at this point. A pair was ready to use at Claremont in the case of a difficult delivery, but because doctors tended to be very conservative with royalty, Croft decided against using the forceps to assist Charlotte at birth. By noon on the 5 November, meconium (faeces from the baby's gut) was found to be leaking from the birth canal – a sign that the baby was in distress.

More than 48 hours after her treacherous labour began, Charlotte delivered a stillborn child on the evening of 5 November. To make matters worse, the child was a boy. Doctors tried in vain to resuscitate the boy; his tiny lungs were inflated, and everything from mustard to rubbing salt, to brandy was put in his mouth. Considering this case with the medical knowledge we have today, it's almost certain the child had been deceased for several hours. However, Princess Charlotte was young, and there seemed no reason why she would not be able to have another child.

After the birth of a child, the mother's uterus should contract to deliver the placenta. However, in Charlotte's case, her uterine contractions were too weak, and it was decided that Sir Croft should remove the placenta by hand. His notes on the case are as such: 'In passing my hand, I met some blood in the uterus but no difficulty until I got to the contract part of the uterus. I afterwards peeled off nearly two-thirds the adhering placenta with considerable facility.'[4]

As was acceptable for the time, a large bandage was placed around Charlotte's stomach. Her pulse was monitored after the removal of the placenta and was deemed to be normal. Charlotte gained her strength back with hot wine, toast, and chicken broth, and her spirits seemed to be improving.

Her physicians turned in for the evening, but by midnight, Charlotte took a turn for the worse. She showed signs of blood loss and complained of a ringing in her ears. She began to vomit and grew extremely restless and had difficulty breathing. It seems likely that Charlotte was bleeding into her uterus, but the bandage around her would have made it hard to detect any enlargement in her abdomen. When Croft was called, he noted that her pulse was rapid and irregular.

In the early morning hours on 6 November 1817, Princess Charlotte passed away. During her post-mortem, the king's sergeant surgeon noted that:

> The child was well formed and weighed nine pounds. Every part of its internal structure was quite sound. The brain and lungs of the mother are normal, but the uterus contained a considerable quantity of coagulated blood and extended as high as the navel, and the hourglass contraction was still apparent.[5]

It is likely that Princess Charlotte died from blood loss rather than childbed fever, a uterine infection would have taken some time to develop. The fact that Charlotte passed so soon after delivery, with the excess amount of blood in her uterus, tells us that she most likely bled to death. Sadly, her life may have been saved had her physicians decided to go ahead with the forceps delivery earlier, or by better post-care following the delivery of the placenta. While the risk of uterine bleeding was understood at the time, the practice of binding the uterus after delivery most likely masked what was happening. Thus, Croft was unable to properly assess the situation.

What makes this story even more dreadful is the fact that Sir Richard Croft was so distraught over the death of Princess Charlotte that he suffered from a deep sense of melancholy. On 13 February 1818, he retired to his bedroom and was later found by a servant girl lying on his back, with a pistol in his hand, aimed at his temple. He was already deceased.

With the death of Princess Charlotte, there remained no heir to the British throne. The death of the princess and her son had eliminated King George III's only legitimate grandchild, and the succession was now in turmoil. All of Charlotte's daughters and daughters-in-law were past their childbearing years, and her three sons remained unmarried.

The second son of the king and queen, Frederick Duke of York and Albany, had already died of heart failure. His neglected wife was childless and died shortly after her husband. The king's third son, William, Duke of Clarence, was wholly devoted to his mistress and saw no need to change anything before the death of Princess Charlotte. Realising any illegitimate children he had could not inherit the throne, William decided to marry. His marriage to Princess Adelaide of Saxe-Meiningen would produce a daughter, but she only lived a few hours. A second daughter born to the couple also died in infancy. With the death of George IV in 1830, William inherited the throne. He was 65 years old. However, seven years later, he died of pneumonia.

The fourth child, Edward, Duke of Kent (Victoria's father), was born in 1767. He was a clever child and at the age of 17 he went to Hanover, Germany, to study. Edward favoured women and money and had an almost obsessive devotion to military affairs. He did, however, marry Princess Victoire in 1818. Victoire became pregnant soon after the wedding, and a daughter was born on the morning of 24 May 1819. She was named Victoria.

Victoria's christening was a month later in the Cupola Room at Kensington Palace, and she was given the name Alexandrina Victoria; she soon became known in the family as Drina.

She was a healthy child who grew up speaking German but also learned English at the age of three. Victoria and her family originally wanted to move back to Germany but decided on a quiet home in Devon called Wallbrook Cottage. Winters in Devon were long and cold, and during the winter of January 1820, the season developed into a rollercoaster of storms. It seemed impossible to keep the house warm no matter how much coal was piled on the grates. Every room in the house was freezing, and all the family members eventually caught a cold. Victoria thankfully recovered quickly, but her father would not fare so well.

In early January, after caring for his horses, Edward came into the home wet and cold and quickly developed a sore throat. Despite feeling terrible, he kept up his social engagements. His wife cared for him with quinine treatments and moved his bed into the warmest room in the house. Dr Wilson (1809–1844), the family physician, began the treatment of applying leeches to Edward's chest on 10 January. Two days later, he took a turn for the worse and began to develop pneumonia, along with chest pain, delirium, and high fever. Sadly, as with Princess Charlotte, the practice of bleeding did him no favours. Dr Wilson's desperate courses of leeching and then cupping undoubtedly weakened him. Cupping involves using a vessel filled with hot air to draw blood to the skin. Cupping was done all over the duke's body, including his head. This much distressed the ladies of the household. One of Victoria's ladies, who was already sceptical of the treatment, said: 'It was too dreadful. There is hardly a spot on his dear body which has not been touched by cupping, blisters, or bleeding.'[6]

Dr William Manton, one of the royal physicians to the king, was summoned to Devon to observe the duke's worsening health. Before he arrived, Edward had more than six pints of blood removed. Normal blood volume for the body is eight pints, but the continuous leeching and blistering removed a small quantity of blood each time. Edward's body could have replaced the lost fluid, but red blood cells take 120 days to grow, and at the end of the alarming number of bleedings, the haemoglobin in his blood would have only been between 40 and 50 per cent of what was needed. In such a feeble state, the infection in his lungs would have been exacerbated and the circulation of his heart and lungs in dire straits. It's almost certain that the antibodies and white blood cells needed to fight his illness were continually being drained by the obsessive bleeding. Dr Manton's therapy likely sped up the timing of Edward's death.

The duke was roused enough to sign his will, before dying on 23 January, just two weeks after he became sick. Years later, Dr Manton was convinced that 'the duke would be borne more depletion',[7] meaning that he should have been bled even more. After the death of the duke, Victoria, her mother, and her siblings, returned to London and were given rooms at Kensington Palace by Prince Leopold, Victoria's uncle. There, Victoria played with her collection of dolls as a child and a music box. She was a bright-eyed and happy child.

Only two months after Victoria was born, her midwife attended the labour of the wife of the Duke of Saxe-Coburg and Saalfeld (1784–1844). On the 26th of August 1819, she gave birth to a boy whom she named Albert (1819–1861). At the birth, the midwife remarked that the infant would make a fine husband for his cousin Victoria.

While growing up at Kensington Palace, Victoria's uncle Leopold had his own plans to manipulate affairs in a new direction as soon as Victoria's succession to the throne was in place. He pressed Victoria with the idea of marriage to his nephew, Albert.

By the age of 17 Victoria was maturing into an intelligent and independent young woman – much to the dismay of her overbearing mother. Leopold invited her cousins Albert (1819–1861) and Ernest (1818–1893) to London. Victoria was not overly impressed with Albert, who had a hard time staying awake past 10 pm, even when at important gatherings. She told her uncle, 'I may not have the feeling for him which is requisite to ensure happiness.'[8]

Following the death of her uncle, King William IV on 20 June 1837, less than one month after her 18th birthday, Victoria became queen of England. She demonstrated strong sense and excellent poise and accepted Lord Melbourne (1779–1848) as her prime minister. Her uncle Leopold continued to write to her about Albert, but she had already established her independence and claimed that: 'my poor uncle seems to be out of humour because I have not asked his advice, but it is my uncle who seems to imagine that his mission is to rule everywhere. I, myself, see no need for that.'[9]

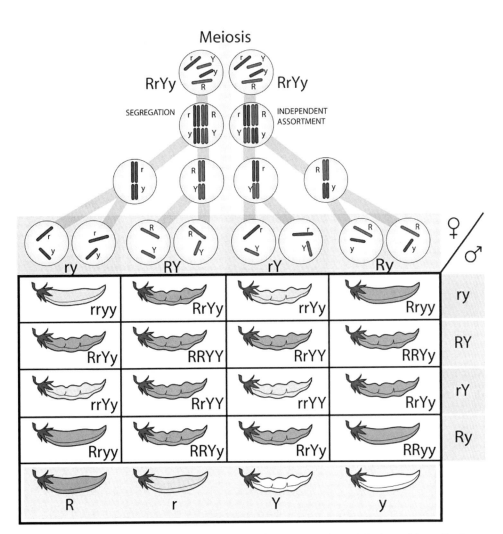

Mendel's Law of Heredity. (https://biologydictionary.net/mendels-law-of-heredity/)

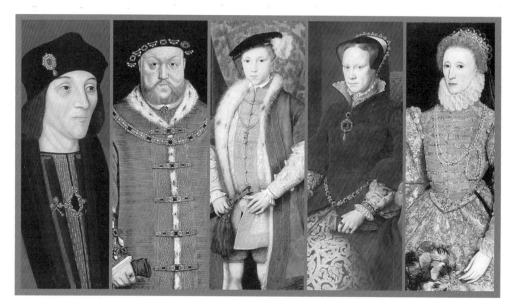

Tudor Monarchy. (https://www.bbc.co.uk/teach/school-radio/history-tudors-image-gallery/zk3fpg8)

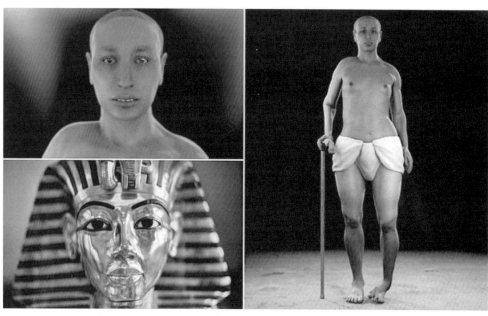

King Tutankhamun. (https://www.foxnews.com/science/is-this-the-face-of-tutankhamun)

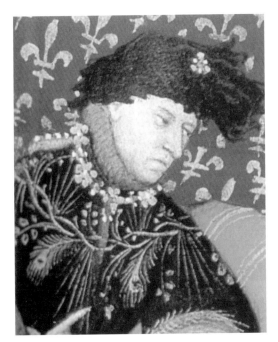
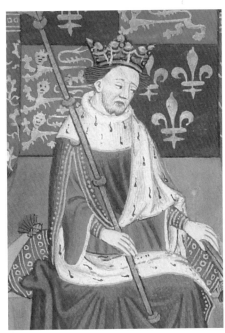

Charles VI of France. (https://www.ancientpages.com/2016/01/22/charles-vi-france-king-made-glass/)

Henry VI of England. (https://en.wikipedia.org/wiki/Henry_VI_of_England)

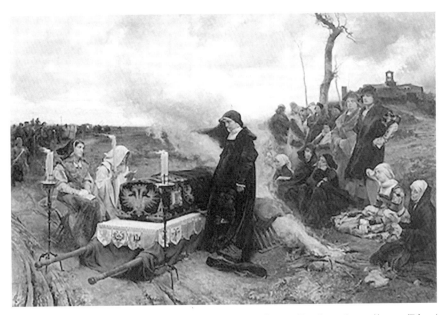

Juana the Mad and Her Husband's Casket. (https://onthetudortrail.com/Blog/2010/11/13/grief-and-coffins-was-juana-of-castile-really-mad/)

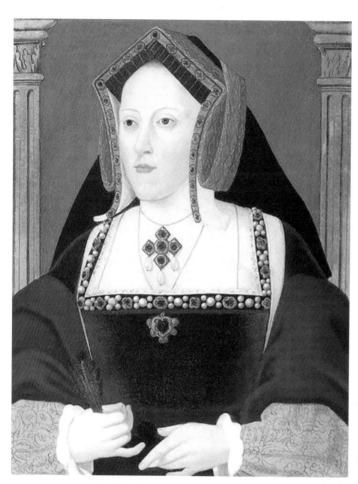

Katherine of Aragon. (https://www.biography.com/royalty/catherine-of-aragon)

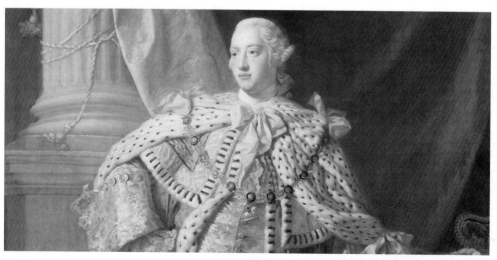

Mad King George of England. (https://brewminate.com/mad-king-george-and-his-doctor/)

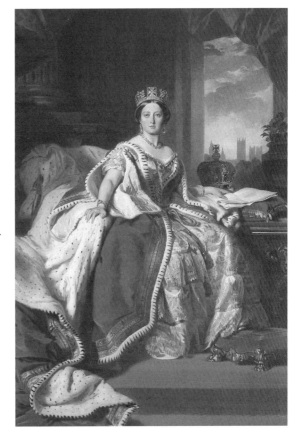

Right: Queen Victoria of
England. (https://www.popsugar.
com/celebrity/queen-victoria-
facts-44002237)

Below left: Prince Leopold of
England. (https://www.pinterest.
com/pin/99571841739661320/)

Below right: Tsarina Alexandra
and Tsarevich Alexei of
Russia. (https://oldspirituals.
com/2015/04/12/rasputin-
influence-romanovs/)

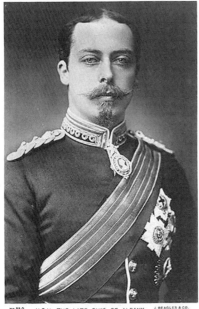

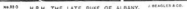

No.920   H.R.H. THE LATE DUKE OF ALBANY.   J. BEAGLES & CO.

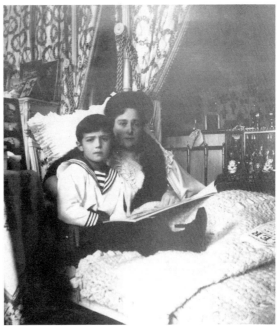

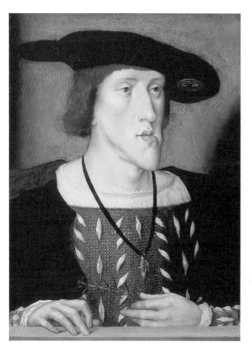 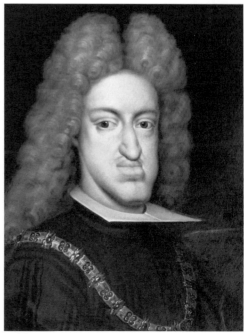

Above left: Charles V and the Hapsburg Jaw. (https://en.wikipedia.org/wiki/Charles_V,_Holy_Roman_Emperor)

Above right: Charles II of Spain. (https://www.thefamouspeople.com/profiles/charles-ii-of-spain-32195.php)

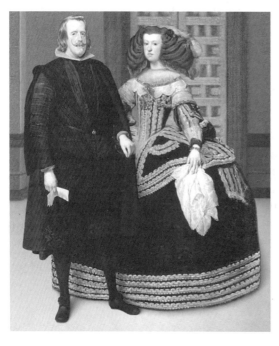

Philip IV and his Niece-Bride Mariana of Austria. (https://noloseytu.blogspot.com/2015/11/mariana-de-austria-y-felipe-iv.html)

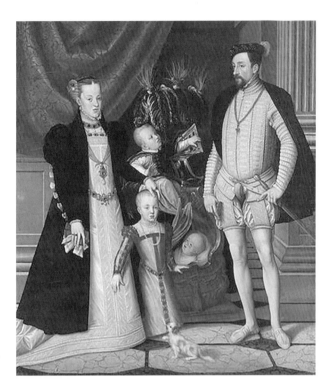

Anna of Austria and
her Uncle-Husband
Philip II of Spain. (https://
s3.amazonaws.com/
s3.timetoast.com/public/
uploads/photo/13063873/
image/6a5d54bf5f2770064
b652f7fff18918e)

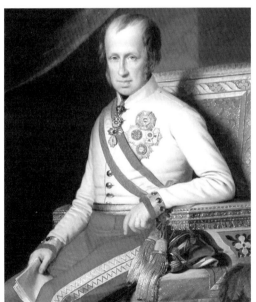

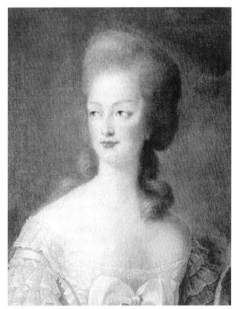

Above left: Ferdinand I of Austria. (https://en.wikipedia.org/wiki/Ferdinand_I_of_
Austria)

Above right: Queen Marie Antoinette of France. (https://allthatsinteresting.com/
habsburg-jaw)

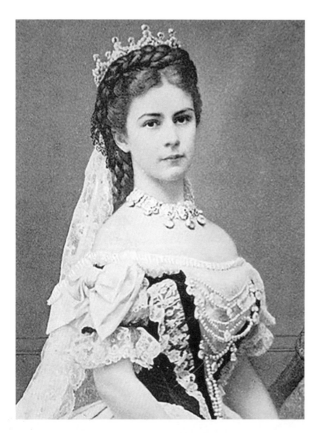

Left: Empress Sisi of Austria. (https://en.wikipedia.org/wiki/Empress_Elisabeth_of_Austria)

Below: King Ludwig II of Bavaria. (https://en.wikipedia.org/wiki/Ludwig_II_of_Bavaria)

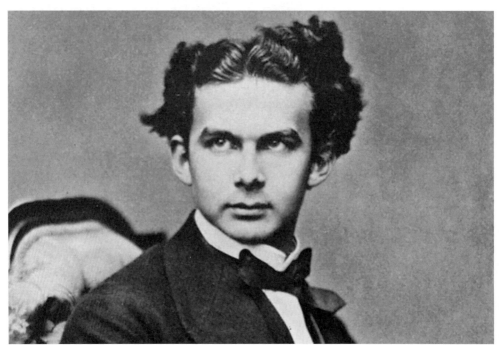

Two years after Victoria's coronation, Leopold once again suggested that Albert visit England, but by this time, Albert too, was getting a bit tired of the pressure. He agreed to visit London but only to put an end to the idea with a 'quiet but firm resolution'. However, Albert's plan to abandon the idea of marriage went awry when he again saw his cousin. And Victoria seemed just as smitten by him.

Albert had grown from a sickly-looking boy into a very handsome young man, and within hours of meeting again, he had completely swept his cousin, the queen, off her feet.

'Albert really is quite charming and so excessively handsome!' she claimed. Three days later, Victoria told Albert that she would be only 'too happy if he would consent to what I wished', meaning marriage. It seemed that Albert had forgotten about Victoria's 'incredible stubbornness', which had turned him off at their prior meetings. The two fell deeply in love with one another.[10]

On 10 February 1840, Queen Victoria married her cousin Albert. She wrote in her diary: 'Oh, to feel I was, and am, loved by such an angel as Albert was too great a delight to describe.'[11]

Victoria had hoped to wait before having children, but because neither she nor Albert had an idea of how to avoid pregnancy, she conceived one month after their wedding. Her pregnancy was uneventful; she ate well and didn't have to endure the bleeding that went along with a royal pregnancy as her aunt had to endure.

On 21 November of that year, after a twelve-hour labour, Victoria delivered a premature baby girl named Victoria Adelaide Mary Louisa (1840–1901), who was nicknamed Vicky. Victoria soon learned she rather disliked babies, saying they looked like frogs, but both Vicky's parents did find great joy in her. The queen also never breastfed her babies, though it was not uncommon for royals to forgo this. When Vicky was born prematurely, her wet nurse had to be sent for unexpectedly, and she was given supplementary food until her arrival. Because Queen Victoria refused to nurse, she increased her chances of another pregnancy. Doctors didn't understand at the time that breastfeeding was a reliant contraceptive, and the queen was quick to be over the process of lactation.

With the end of lactation came Victoria's menses, and her second child was conceived only three months after the birth of Vicky. Edward (1841–1910) (later Edward VII) was born on 9 November 1841. Because her disdain for nursing had not changed, a wet nurse was called; Victoria soon became pregnant again and delivered a daughter, Alice (1843–1878), seventeen months after the birth of Edward. In a letter written to Vicky later in life, the queen said:

> What made me so miserable was to have the first two years of married life utterly spoilt by this occupation of pregnancy. I could enjoy nothing, not travel about, or go about with dear Papa. If I had waited a year, as I hope you will, it would have been very different.[12]

While Victoria did feel some joy at the birth of her first son, Edward was soon looked at as being rather dull and having temper tantrums. Several children followed Edward: Alfred (1844–1900), Helena (1846–1923), Louise (1848–1939), Arthur (1850–1942), Leopold (1853–1944), and lastly, Beatrice (1857–1944). The queen's pregnancies were uncomfortable, and her deliveries painful. Four of her daughters were married in their late teens, but Beatrice stayed at home with her mother until the age of 28.

Beatrice and Alice were the only two of Victoria's daughters to carry the gene for haemophilia, and Leopold was the only boy to suffer from the disease. Leopold's delivery, on 7 April 1853, was unremarkable. The queen was given chloroform by her doctor, which was very controversial, because at the time, any pain relief from childbirth was seen as a 'decoy of Satan'.[13] But Victoria found that anaesthesia in childbirth was 'soothing, quieting and delightful beyond measure'.

Although Leopold was described as a jolly baby, Victoria suffered depression worse than after the birth of her other children. Disputes arose, and Albert said she would collapse into: 'a continuance of hysterics for more than an hour … traces of which remained for more than 24 hours'.[14]

Victoria paid very little attention to Leopold who was left in the complete care of a wet nurse. It was only when he began to walk, that it was noticed he bruised easily. He was soon diagnosed with haemophilia and those that were against the use of chloroform blamed it for Leopold's condition. It seemed that the queen's attitudes to certain members of her family were incredibly unbalanced. While she ended up growing close to Leopold, she had total disregard for her eldest, Edward, who was heir to the throne. She regarded him as being slow minded and was entirely disliked by her.

It seems she still had sour words for Leopold even though they had a better relationship. She described him as a chronic invalid who was a terrible speaker and unattractive because of his haemorrhaging disorder. 'He bruises as much as ever but, unberufen (German for 'touch wood') 1,000 times, is free from any at present, but holds himself still as badly as ever and is very ugly. I think uglier than he ever was.'[15]

She also wrote:

> he still bruises as much as ever, but he has unberufen, not had any accidents as of late. He is tall but holds himself worse than ever and is a very common looking child, very pale in the face, clever but an oddity and not an engaging child though amusing.[16]

In describing his height, the queen said:

> Leopold was the smallest when born, and he is the tallest of his age of any of you and the ugliest. An ugly baby is a very nasty object.[17]

Victoria seemed so ashamed of Leopold that she left him behind when the rest of the family would go on holiday, saying:

> Leopold still has such constant bad accidents that it would be very troublesome indeed to have him here. He walks shockingly and dreadfully awkward, holds himself badly as ever, and his manners are despairing, as well as his speech, which is quite dreadful.[18]

And just as she consistently lamented Leopold's looks, she became obsessed with Prince Edward's perceived stupidity. She described her son as 'feeble',[19] and his childhood was filled with education lessons from 8 am to 7 pm, six days a week.

* * * *

In 1861, Prince Albert fell ill and passed on the 14 December. The cause was either typhoid or a stomach cancer that had gone undetected. No postmortem exam was performed.

Victoria, only 42 years old, was completely devastated by the loss of her husband: 'I who felt, when those bold arms clasped and held tight in the sacred hours of the night, the world seemed only to be ourselves, that nothing could part us. I felt so very secure.'

The queen refused to open Parliament for five years and spent each night with a horrific deathbed picture of Albert on her pillow next to her while she clutched his nightshirt in her arms. Each morning, she had hot shaving water brought to his old rooms and each day his unused chamber pot was to be scoured.

Young Prince Leopold, who was in the French Riviera at the time, was deeply upset by his father's death. Despite this, he still managed to be a carefree and prankster of a child. He would often poke fun at his own blood disorder and once at breakfast ran into the room with a handkerchief soaked in red, saying he had had a tooth pulled. After much fussing over him and attention, he revealed that it was only red paint on the cloth and not blood.

Despite his joking manner, Prince Leopold suffered greatly from his disorder, as is apparent in his letters to his sister, Louisa. On 10 June 1870, he wrote:

> I go on as usual, suffering frightfully. At this moment, I am in agony of pain; my knee gets worse daily, and I get more desperate daily. If this continues long, I shall soon be driven to Bedlam or Hanwell, where I shall be fortunately able to terminate a wretched existence by knocking out my brains (if I have any) on the walls; that is the brightest vision that I can picture to myself as a future. But I must stop on account of the awful pain which is torturing me.

While there was no treatment for Leopold's disease, his physicians did take great care in trying to help him. Sir William Jenner (1815–1898), the queen's personal physician, cared for Leopold from 1861 until his death. John Wickham Legg (1843–1921), an understudy of Jenner's, also personally served Leopold from 1866–1867. He kept a close relationship with him, not only as a physician but as a source of comfort. In contrast to many doctors of the time, Dr Legg warned against bloodletting. He also warned against any surgeries as well as damp or cold climates. He believed that those with the disorder should spend as much time as possible in warm climates and urged Leopold to do this.

In 1877, at age 24, Leopold became one of his mother's private secretaries and was given more access to state papers than Edward ever was. He became his mother's trusted advisor and intermediary between her and leading politicians. In 1881, Leopold was made Duke of Albany and began the process of looking for a bride. In mid-April 1882, Leopold married Princess Helena of Waldeck (1861–1922), a sister to the Dutch queen.

Shortly after his wedding, Leopold suffered a serious episode of bleeding after slipping on an orange peel. At the birth of his daughter

Alice (1883–1981) in February of 1883, Leopold was bedridden. The following year, he was sent by his doctors to Cannes to escape the severe cold of the March winter; unfortunately, he fell down a staircase at his hotel which resulted in a brain haemorrhage. He died hours later. The queen said of her son's death: 'my darling Leopold had died at 3.30 this morning quite suddenly in his sleep from the breaking of a blood vessel in his head. I am utterly crushed.'[20]

Queen Victoria ruled over one of the largest empires the world had ever seen. More cities were founded in her name than for Alexander the Great. But she also carried the deadly haemophilia gene, and there was only limited scientific understanding of the disorder at the time. And because of this lack of understanding, Victoria's grandchildren would continue to spread the gene that would contribute to the history of the world.

Haemophilia, by etymological definition, means 'love of blood' and was not completely understood after Queen Victoria passed. And in order to understand the disease, we must understand the dynamics behind the clotting of blood. Like most mammals, the human cardiovascular system works at high pressure, carrying blood to every organ via blood vessels and capillaries. In our lives, some sort of injury involving the cardiovascular system is almost inevitable. This could be a minor injury with only slight damage to a few capillaries, or it could be a major trauma that leads to the breaking of a major blood vessel. In any event, our cardiovascular system is incredibly complex, and the medical world has taken considerable time to fully understand how human blood clots. Some physicians believed it was a defect in the blood vessels, and some even thought it was the male equivalent of monthly menstruation. In 1891, Sir Almoth Wright (1861–1947), an English medical scientist, discovered that the blood of one plagued with haemophilia took longer to clot than that of a someone without the condition.

Scientists already understood that blood contained a protein called fibrinogen. When a clot formed, it was converted into a fibrin network, pushing against any hole in which blood could escape. Today we know that for fibrinogen to turn to fibrin, the enzyme thrombin is needed. But it was the origin of thrombin that remained the most complicated part of the process, and it took quite some time before the understanding of blood clotting would be fully understood. Many factors come into play to form thrombin, such as blood platelets, enzymes, prothrombin, and other factors. If even one factor is compromised in this chain of events, serious complications can arise during the body's attempt to clot the blood. This kink in the chain of events to form thrombin surfaces is the basis of haemophilia.

While the disease is hereditary and infants are born with it, they do not seem to bleed any more during birth than other babies. However, once the child begins to become mobile, they may bruise easily – crawling can cause bleeding into the knees for example. Those with the disease can easily bleed anywhere, from the mouth to the intestines, to the brain, skin, or joints. Bleeding in the joints is relatively common and incredibly debilitating as it causes swelling, restricted movement, and a fever. The blood eventually clots in the joint but is then replaced by fibrous tissue, leading to deformities. Parents of children may notice that their baby is frightened by even the smallest jarring motion.

During the nineteenth century, records show that others who shared the same affliction as Leopold and haemorrhage terribly after small accidents. Tradesman could die from a simple prick from a nail, while others may have died from accidents involving animals or their farming equipment.

Prince Leopold's haemophilia was not only serious but incurable. The unpredictable disease put great demands on him and his parents. And unfortunately for him, the treatment of the disease was often worse than the disease itself. Although Dr Legg may have advised against bleeding, the practice of treating haemophilia by being bled was still advisable by many doctors. The application of leeches, cupping, or any other deliberate opening of veins would have been disastrous.

* * * *

The final years of Queen Victoria's life were rather tragic and undoubtedly took their toll on the Monarch. In April of 1900, her eldest son, the Prince of Wales, was shot by a protester in Belgium. Her eldest daughter, Vicky, was diagnosed with breast cancer that had spread to her spine and kept her in considerable pain. In August of that same year, her son Alfred died from throat cancer. Alfred was one of the queen's favourite children, and upon hearing of his death, she wrote: 'Oh! God! My poor darling Alfie gone too! My third grown-up child. It is hard at 81!'

Only a few weeks later, Victoria learned that her grandson, Prince Christian (1876–1900), was stricken with enteric fever, and on Christmas Day, Lady Jane Churchill (1826–1900), the queen's most trusted friend, had passed away.

Understandably, Victoria suffered greatly from these losses. She began to lose weight and lost her appetite and stayed confined to her wheelchair. She had been on the throne for sixty-four years and the future of her reign seemed near its end, however she seemed reluctant to fully accept her coming demise. As her illness progressed, she asked her physician, 'Sir James, 'I should like to live a little longer as I have still a few things to settle.'

On 17 January 1901, the queen suffered from a series of strokes and her family was summoned to her bedside. While barely conscious, she continued to say to her physician, 'Sir James, I'm very ill.'

She passed away on 22 January, with her children and grandchildren by her side. Little did she know that one of those grandchildren would give birth to a little boy who would suffer terribly from the same blood disorder as his great-uncle Leopold.

Chapter Nine

Tsarevich Alexei's Royal Disease and the End of the Russian Monarchy

In early June of 1872, Alexandra Feodorovna (1872–1919) was born as the Princess of Hesse and Rhine, a duchy part of the German empire. Her mother, Alice, was the second daughter of Queen Victoria, making Alexandra – nicknamed Alix – Victoria's granddaughter.

Alix's childhood was not immune to disease and death. Her brother, Friedrich (1871–1873), would die of Victoria's dreaded disease at only two years old.

On 14 December 1878, when Alix was just six, her mother died of diphtheria. She also lost her younger sister Marie (1874–1878). Queen Victoria took Alix under her wing and became very protective of her, and the two grew very close.

In early 1892, Alix suffered the loss of her other parent when her father, Grand Duke Louis IV (1837–1892), died of a heart attack. She was struck deeply by her father's passing and could not speak of him for years without collapsing in tears.

Queen Victoria wanted to secure a good future for her favourite granddaughter and tried to find her the perfect love match but realised, after several failed attempts, that Alix had her own strength of character.

In 1884, during her first visit to Russia, Alix met and fell in love with Nicholas, heir to the Russian throne. The couple overcame the obstacles of a difference of faith as Alix considered a conversion to Russian Orthodox from Lutheran. In November of 1894, she married Nicholas, and the two became Tsar and Tsarina of Russia.

The couple promptly started their family, giving birth to four healthy daughters in a span of eight years, but because the throne could only be passed to a male heir, Alix felt building pressure to give birth to a son. She bathed in the holy waters of Serafin and prayed for a male heir to be sent to her.

Her wish was granted, as her long-awaited heir was born on 4 August 1904 at Peterhof Palace in St Petersburg. The first heir to the Russian throne since the 17th century was born at a healthy eight pounds, and cities across the country celebrated with cannons, gunfire, church bells and flags. Alexei Nikolaevich, Sovereign Heir Tsarevich, Grand Duke of Russia (1904–1918), was a chubby baby with blonde hair and blue eyes and was adored by his sisters. Although he appeared to be healthy, there was concern when the umbilical cord was cut, and he bled for forty-eight hours as the blood would not clot.

The family's happiness over his birth was short-lived when Alexei suffered his first episode of what would become a painful and debilitating disease. It was feared he had inherited the 'English Disease' from his mother. An entry from the diary of Nicholas II tells of his anxiety when his son was just 6 weeks old:

> Alix and I have been very much worried. A haemorrhage began this morning without the slightest cause from the navel of our small Alexei. It lasted but a few hours but a few interruptions until evening. We had to call the surgeon, who, at 7 pm, applied a bandage, and the child was remarkably quiet. He seemed merry, but it was a dreadful thing to have through such anxiety.[1]

It took three days for the bleeding to stop, and fear grew in the family. As Alexei learned to stand up, crawl and walk, he would stumble as babies do. Little bumps and bruises would turn dark blue in a few hours as his blood failed to clot under his skin, and the fears that Alexei had inherited haemophilia from his mother turned into reality, a tragedy that would change the course of Russian history.

Alexei's secret was hidden from the world as the family stayed at their home, Tsarskoe Selo. The palace, built by Catherine I, was kept under heavy guard to protect the royal family. Inside the palace, the family lived a fairly routine life, with Nicky rising at the same time every day, eating breakfast, and going to his study. Alix spent her time reading and writing letters to her friends, curled up with her Scottish Terrier, Eira. Each day before the children began their studies, they were given a quick exam by the court physician, Dr Botkin (1865–1918), to be sure all was well. Alexei was also under the direct care of Dr Vladimir De Revenko (1879–1936).

Alexei was a happy child and the centre of the family's attention: 'Alexei was the centre of the united family, the focus of all its hopes and affections. His sisters worshipped him, and he was his parent's pride and joy. When he was well, the palace was transformed. Everything and everyone was bathed in sunshine.'[2]

As Alexei began to walk, his tumbles caused large swellings on his limbs. At one time, he fell on his forehead, and his face became so swollen that his eyes were sealed shut, and it took almost three weeks for the swelling to subside.

Medically speaking, a nightmare was brewing inside the boy's body. His blood did not clot normally, so every minor bump or bruise would rupture the tiny blood vessels beneath his skin. The blood would then seep into the surrounding muscles and tissues, where it would eventually cause a haematoma – sometimes the size of a grapefruit. Small scratches didn't seem to be that serious as they were immediately wrapped with tight bandages to pinch off the blood, allowing the scratch to heal. But if Alexei suffered cuts in the mouth or nose which could not be bandaged, he was in danger. At one point, he almost died as the result of a simple nosebleed.

Alexei's disease was not only terrifying, but it was incredibly painful. Because the blood would pool in his joints, it put pressure on the nerves causing terrible pain. The boy often cried to his mother that he could not bend his knees or elbows because it hurt so much. While morphine was available as pain relief, his parents were too afraid to let doctors give it to him, and so his only relief was when he would pass out from the pain. The blood inside Alexei's joints destroyed the bone, cartilage and tissue and changed the formation of the bone. This caused his limbs to lock into position.

Doctors prescribed exercise and massage, but this also risked another haemorrhage. Heavy iron orthopaedic devices and hot mud baths were given to straighten his limbs. These treatments caused Alexei to spend days in bed recovering, where he was watched by nurses around the clock.

Alexei was also appointed two male bodyguards to keep him from hurting himself. Derevenko and Nagorny, sailors from the Imperial Navy, were calm and patient with him. They would often assist him in stretching his limbs and moving about carefully.

The effects of haemophilia seemed to come in waves, and Alexei was able to lead a relatively normal life in-between flare-ups. He was a mischievous child who would break into his sisters' room and disturb their studies and crash dinner parties by crawling under the table, grabbing the feet of the guests. He knew he was important and welcomed the fuss the public made over him, especially the plethora of gifts he received. However, Alexei also had a reputation being a bit of a bratty child, and while his parents warned him against certain activities, these seemed to be the very ones he gravitated towards. He seemed to favour dangerous activities, perhaps because he wasn't allowed to ride bikes and play tennis like other children. One time, Alexei found a bike and rode it around the palace as guards attempted to capture him. His parents showered him with safer toys, such as trains and toy soldiers, to keep him busy.

At one point, after standing on a chair, Alexei slipped and banged his knee on the corner of a desk. The following day he was unable to walk, and subcutaneous haemorrhaging started. The swelling in his knee spread down his leg, making his distended skin hard and painful to the touch. Alix stayed by his bedside and tried everything she could to alleviate her son's pain. His father's attempts at distracting him with humour were not helpful, and when his sisters came to visit, Alexei hardly recognised them.

Black circles surrounded his eyes, and the doctors grew more concerned as he began to run a fever. He cried in agony, wrapped in his mother's arms.

Pierre Gilliard (1879–1962), Alexei's tutor, recalls: 'Think of the torture of that mother, an impotent witness to her son's martyrdom in those hours of anguish. A mother who knew that she, herself, was the cause of that suffering, that she had transmitted that terrible disease against which human science was powerless.'

* * * *

We know that haemophilia is a blood clotting deficiency transmitted by women, due to the sex-linked mendelian pattern, and although women carry the defect, there is scarce, if any, history of a woman having the disorder. Haemophilia doesn't always affect every male in a family, as families may not even know they are affected by it until it passes to a son. Parents can be unaware that a female child carries the gene until she goes on to have her own children. The disease follows no racial or geographical pattern and is consistent throughout the world. Forty per cent of people with the condition today have no traceable history of the disease in their family, as it can go hidden for generations. The gene also seems to change and mutate without any explanation as to why.

It is assumed that in Queen Victoria's case, the haemophilia was a result of spontaneous mutation and her son Leopold suffered because of that. It is unknown whether Alix was privy to her uncle Leopold's suffering, but we know that her mother Alice, and likely her aunt, Beatrice, were carriers of the disease.

Frederick, or Frittie, was Alix's brother who inherited the disease from their mother. He was diagnosed only a few months before his death, and he suffered a cut on his ear and bled for three days despite the application of bandages. A few months later, in May of 1873,

Frittie was playing with his brother in their mother's bedroom. During the play, Frittie tumbled out of a window and fell 20ft. He died only hours later of a brain haemorrhage but may have survived this fall if he had not been a haemophiliac. The sons of Alix's aunt Irene (1866–1953) were also affected by the disease as her son Henry (1900–1904) died at age 4 and his brother, Waldemar, at age 56 (1889–1945).

The gene pattern had already been discovered in 1803, and it was cautioned that a family with the gene should not be allowed to marry. So, Alix must have known that her family was affected and yet seemed almost shocked that Alexei inherited it. While the gene pattern was understood by doctors, the details of it were not discussed in the royal courts of Europe, making haemophilia the gap between royal families and everyday life at the time. And even with some understanding of the disorder, the main goal of royal families was to produce a male heir and not consider anything that may complicate that.

The Tsarina must have felt tremendous pressure not only to birth a son but to protect him at all costs. During the course of history, the death of a child was almost expected, and if that child was a male heir, disaster could easily set in. After the birth of four girls, Nicholas was understandably frustrated not only with the situation but with his wife. So, when Alexei was finally born, it was seen as not only the blessing of a son but the blessing of their marriage.

Like every child, Alexei looked to his mother to ease his pain, and when it came to the pain of haemophilia, there was nothing Alix could do. She looked for answers in the Russian Orthodox Church, as they had a strong belief in the power of healing through prayer. Alix continued to plead and beg God to keep her son safe, and never lost her faith that He would help.

Alix shared a close relationship with one of her ladies-in-waiting, Anna Vyrubova (1884–1964), who would soon tell her of the great mystic Rasputin (1869–1914), who, as far as Alix was concerned, was the answer to her prayers. The mystery of Grigori Rasputin is one that, to this day, is still associated with the Russian royal family, particularly the Tsarina.

Rasputin was born in January of 1869, in a small village in what is now Siberia. His childhood is one that is filled with a lot of mystery and reliable sources don't have much information on. He was likely not formally educated and may have been an unruly youth, getting caught up in theft and drinking.

He was married in 1887 and had three children that survived to adulthood. In 1897 he left his family and children for reasons that are still unclear today. He had developed an interest in religion and went on a pilgrimage. It's possible he was escaping prosecution for horse theft, and others claim he went on a pilgrimage because he had visions of the Virgin Mary. After a stay at St Nicholas Monastery in Verkhoturye, Rasputin was transformed. He may have learned to read and write here but he then left the monastery, claiming their way of life was too intimidating.

He returned to his home a changed man and his life took a bizarre turn. He dressed poorly and bathed very little, rarely changing his clothes. He was said to be very dishevelled with dirty hair and fingernails and he omitted a terrible body odor. He also became a vegetarian and swore off alcohol along with devoting much of his life to prayer.

Despite his dirty, unkempt appearance, he developed a circle of followers – many of them women who found him very attractive. He was called the miracle worker and his attendants were convinced that he was a holy man. Secret prayer meetings were held with his followers that became the subject of suspicion that possibly included singing strange songs and participating in sexual orgies and self-harm.

People who spent time around Rasputin claimed it was his eyes that made him stand out. Large, bright, and brilliant blue, they seemed to entrance even those who wholly despised him. His eyes drew people in with their hypnotic stare, radiating magnetism when he spoke to both men and women. Secret prayer meetings were held with his followers that became the subject of suspicion that possibly included sexual orgies and self harm.

One visitor to his prayer meetings stated:

'Rasputin had tremendous hypnotic power. I felt as if some energy were pouring heat, like a warm current, into my whole being.'

Rasputin used his charm to seduce people, especially women. People referred to him as 'a starlet, a man of God who lived in poverty and solitude, offering himself as a guide to the other moments of suffering and turmoil.'

It was this hold on people that would eventually make him such a big part of the Russian Monarchy.

His first meeting with the royal family wouldn't be until November of 1905, where he met Tsar Nicholas at Peterhof Palace. Nicholas felt immediately that he and Alix had made the acquaintance of a man of God. The following year he returned and met with the royal children, and the family became convinced that he possessed the power to further heal Alexei. Much of this belief stemmed from Alix who witnessed Rasputin's healing power on more than one occasion. Alix developed a very intense attachment to Rasputin and he soon became an everyday member of the family.

In the spring of 1907, he was asked to heal Alexei, who had suffered yet another haemorrhage. He miraculously stropped bleeding the next morning.

In the summer of 1912, on a shared carriage ride with Anna Vyrubova, Alix and Alexei went for a breath of fresh air, but the bumpy ride caused Alexei to complain of pains in his legs and stomach. By the time they arrived home, Alexei was in a considerable amount of pain.

Dr Botkin found a haemorrhage in the boy's thigh and groin, and after consulting with other court doctors, was still overwhelmed by how quickly Alexei's condition deteriorated. Excerpts from Nicholas's diary from that fateful fall of 1912:

The days between the 6th and 10th were the worst. The poor darling suffered intensely. The pains came in spasms and occurred every quarter of an hour. His high temperature made him delirious night and day. He would sit up in the bed, and every movement would bring the pain on again. He hardly slept at all, had not even the strength to pray, and kept repeating, 'Lord, have mercy on me'.

Alexei's wails of pain were constant, and many servants and courtiers would stuff cotton in their ears to stifle his cries. During this time, Alix stayed with her son by his bed the entire time, as he lay half-conscious with a pale face and his body contorted. He had dark circles under his eyes that were rolled back in his head. Nicky tried to relieve his wife but would burst into tears as soon as he saw his son in such agony. At one point, Alexei asked his mother if the pain would be gone should he die.

On top of trying to ease his suffering, the family fought to keep his illness from the public. But eventually, this was almost impossible as things began to leak to the press about Alexei's health. In London, the *Daily Mail* claimed he had been wounded in a bomb attack before the family regretfully finally let the public know that Alexei was ill – but they didn't reveal the nature of the illness. The country of Russia prayed for their heir day and night.

When it appeared that things could not get any worse for Alexei, his mother called on Rasputin in desperation. She asked Anna, her lady, to message him in Siberia and ask him to pray for Alexei. The following night Alix got a telegram from him assuring her that Alexei would live.

The next morning his bleeding stopped.

The Tsar claimed it was because the boy was given holy communion the night before. Alexei's doctors had no explanation for the sudden turning point in his health but felt there must be some medical reasoning. And it's entirely possible that there was.

After a long period of time, a haemophiliac may stop bleeding on their own. Anaemia in the brain would likely cause fainting, which often happened in Alexei's case. Along with fainting would come a drop in blood pressure, which would cause the bleeding to eventually stop. Today, things are never allowed to get to such a dire point as there is medication that will quickly stop the bleeding.

However, one thing Rasputin said in his letter to Alix was to 'not let the doctors fuss over him so much'. Surely, Alexei must have felt increased stress with the constant probing and temperature taking from his physicians. The poking and pressing on his body possibly could have dislodged any clot that was beginning to form. Is it possible that once the doctors did cease their intervention, Alexei's body was able to heal naturally? The amount of stress in his body may have decreased once his mother received the telegram from Rasputin. If the stress in his mother's body visibly lifted, Alexei's own stress may have done the same if we consider how much he relied on his mother for comfort.

Alix firmly believed that Rasputin was from the hand of God and felt that her son was safe in his care. And, slowly, Alexei did recover. His left leg was drawn up against his chest for a month before doctors could get it moving again, and it would be up to a year before he could walk normally.

In 1915 another amazing 'healing' by Rasputin occurred when Alexei got a bloody nose that bled for two days; Rasputin was called back to the palace and, after a simple laying on of hands, was able to get the bleeding to stop, and Alexei recovered.

Rasputin also made Alexei's four sisters feel at ease around him. He wrote letters to the girls when he was away, forming a tight bond with them. But there was also some questionable activity on his part, as he was often seen with the girls when they were only in their nightclothes. The girl's governess claimed that he would often sit at the girls' bedsides, talking with them and caressing them. The governess spoke up and Alix fired her before she could take her story to the authorities.

Rumours soon began to spread that Rasputin not only seduced the four grand duchesses, but the Tsarina herself. These rumours were fuelled by several letters written by Alix to Rasputin. Offensive cartoons depicting sexual acts between the mystic healer, the Tsarina, and her daughters were soon circulated. Much to the dismay of Alix, Nicholas ordered that Rasputin leave St Petersburg.

Rumours about the family's relationship with Rasputin continued until he was murdered in December of 1916. The four grand duchesses were reported to have been visibly upset by the news of his murder and found comfort in one another.

It will never be known whether these miraculous healings of Alexei Romanov were acts of God delivered through the hand of Rasputin, or simply his body trying to heal itself. Unfortunately, no one could save Alexei and his family from their untimely demise.

In February of 1917, the Imperial family was arrested, and Nicholas II abdicated the throne. They were kept in isolation at the Ipatiev House, the house of a merchant in Yekaterinburg. Alexei continued to deteriorate while being held and, from March of 1918, spent his final weeks in a wheelchair.

On 17 July 1918, the Tsarevich was murdered at the age of 13 by Bolshevik secret police, along with the rest of his family. The boy died not from his horrific childhood disease, but from a gunshot to the head. As we know, the rest of the Russian Royal Family was also murdered, bringing a permanent end to the Russian monarch.

Chapter Ten

The Habsburgs: A Family Notorious for Inbreeding

The Royal House of Habsburg is one of the most powerful dynasties of Medieval and Renaissance Europe, and they would rule much of Europe for almost six centuries. But aside from their great power, there is another reason for their notoriety. The Royal House of Habsburg is the most notorious European dynasty known for its practices of inbreeding. Powerful though they may have been, their devotion to keeping those royal genes close at hand would also be the reason for their downfall.

The Habsburgs consisted of two branches of the family, the Spanish line, and the Austrian line. These two branches of the family were full of inbred cousins, uncles, and nieces. Brides-to-be were continually used as political pawns to secure the dynasty's wealth, power, and pure bloodline. Of course, at the time, the Habsburgs had no idea that this method of breeding would produce family members with mental and physical deformities, miscarriages, and stillbirths. Four out of ten children born into a Habsburg family died before their first birthday, and only five in ten would make it past their tenth birthday. If we compare these numbers to those of a regular Spanish household living during the same time, only two out of ten children would die before reaching adulthood.

To understand just how inbred the Habsburgs were we need to look at how the empire developed. In the early twelfth century, the Habsburgs began to gain power and wealth and quickly expanded their realm from Switzerland to Austria, Hungary, France, Italy, and Spain.

The history of the Habsburg dynasty begins with the election of Rudolph I (1218–1291)) as king of Germany in 1273, also the first king of the House of Habsburg. Rudolph assigned the Duchy of Austria to his sons, and from that moment, the Habsburg dynasty was also known as the House of Austria. In 1438, the Habsburg Archduke of Austria was elected Holy Roman Emperor.

In 1424, 9-year-old Frederick Habsburg (1415 –1493) would become Fredrick the Duke of Inner Austria upon the death of his father. His uncle, Frederick IV of Tyrol (1382–1439), acted as regent. In 1435, he was declared of age to rule, and the following year, he made a pilgrimage to the Holy Land, which would secure his great reputation.

In 1452, he travelled to Italy to be crowned Holy Roman Emperor, the first since the death of the previous Holy Roman Emperor, Sigismund of Luxembourg (1368 –1437). From that day, The Habsburgs would rule the Holy Roman Empire for the next three-and-a-half centuries.

The beginning of the inbreeding disaster with the Habsburgs started with the grandson of Frederick III, Philip of Burgundy. As we know, Philip married Juana of Castile, who was the product of a marriage of second cousins and would ultimately lose control of her kingdom. Juana and Philip had six children that would be married into other families, taking with them, Juana's twisted genetics.

In 1519, Charles V, son of Juana and Philip, would inherit the Holy Roman Empire from his grandfather, Maximillian, ensuring the unity of the empire with Spain.

He was 16, awkward, and still immature. His father, Ferdinand, had appointed Cardinal Cisneros and Archbishop of Saragossa to oversee things until Charles was of age to rule alone. Offended by this, Charles ordered his servants to bring him a hawk, which he brought into the council room and began to pluck its feathers. As his council members looked on in horror, young Charles accused them of 'plucking me at your good pleasure', alluding to the fact that he felt taken advantage of because of his age. He stated that in the future, 'I shall pluck all of you'.

From childhood, it was assumed that Charles must have had some form of epilepsy as he had several convulsive fits as a boy, but it appears that he grew out of them. Charles was described as having a delicate physique and being of average height. However, one of his most prominent features was his chin, which was noticeably pronounced. Charles suffered from a condition called mandibular prognathism, later known as the 'Habsburg Jaw'. In Charles's case, he was endowed with a thick upper lip and misaligned teeth, which prevented him from fully closing his mouth. He also had difficulty chewing his food and mumbled when he spoke. He was said to almost always have a full beard that somewhat hid the malformation on his face.

It is likely that the inbreeding of his mother's family was the cause of the famous Habsburg Jaw, or at least the start of it. Because of genetic homozygosity – the inheritance of the same defective gene from both parents – the defect for mandibular prognathism came two-fold to affect members of the Habsburg family for centuries. It was more than likely that Charles inherited many of his other life's maladies from his mother as well.

Because there was no knowledge of the effects of intermarriage, Charles went on to marry his first cousin Isabella of Portugal (1503–1539), whose aunt was Charles's mother, Juana. Though they were married to keep the close-knit family even closer, Charles and Isabella fell deeply in love. They have seven children, though only three would reach adulthood, following the high infant mortality rate of the Habsburgs.

Gluttony was a constant issue for the emperor throughout his life and probably contributed to his already poor health. His own doctors and his confessor found Charles's love for food not only dietary abuse but downright sinful. In a 1530 letter from his confessor, it implies that Charles was told:

> not to eat those dishes which are injurious to you. And everyone is aware that fish disagrees with your chest.

Remember that your life is not your own but should be preserved for the sake of others. And if Your Majesty chooses to destroy your own property, you should not endanger what belongs to us.[1]

The letter went on to describe some of the coughing fits the emperor would suffer from.

I write in much distress, for I am informed that your chest is sometimes heard farther off than your tongue. I once wished Your Majesty to do some penance for your sins. But if you change this injunction into a firm resistance against gluttony, it will be to you as meritorious as flint and scrounge.[2]

Though he was warned not to eat anything spicy or to indulge in seafood, the emperor did both, nonetheless. He continued to put on weight and found he could never sleep more than four hours a night. Charles V also suffered greatly from several attacks of gout, many of which he wrote about in his memoirs. In 1538 he was forced to miss a visit with Pope Paul III (1468–1549) because of his gout pain. In 1543, he had to suspend a trip to Diest. His attacks of gout seemed to interfere with a lot of his schedule, leaving a fair amount of business unattended, which often led to melancholy.

In 1545, Venetian Ambassador Bernardo Navagero (1507–1565) wrote: 'The poor prince has aroused the compassion of all who have seen him, such as his poor health, feebleness and pale colouring.'[3]

As Charles's health continued to fail, he carried a walking stick to support him when he wasn't carried around by litter. He wore a sling around his neck, and his fingers appeared crippled. Other than rest, there wasn't a remedy that would help alleviate the emperor's discomfort. But as the times dictated, there was the usual complicated regimen of medications, one being a mix of drachm of rhubarb, mushroom, and cassia oil. Perhaps because he was desperate to feel better, Charles would take the advice of almost any quack doctor that offered it.

Several of the emperor's misfortunes were noted in the letters of William Van Male, a companion and secretary of Charles. On 13 January 1551, he wrote:

> For these last two months, I have heard nothing except bilious and melancholic humours, phlebotomy, potions, pills, and things of that sort and usually the very dirge of mortals. Meanwhile, from this great congregation of physicians, so far, no one has gained a true knowledge. First, it was announced to be nephritis, then an abscess in the kidney, then a collection of symptoms that cloud in the cloaca.[4]

In the early part of 1553, the English Ambassador wrote this about the emperor after visiting with him:

> I've never seen the emperor so nigh gone, never so dead in the face, his hand never so lean, pale, and wan. His eyes that were won't to be full of life when all the rest had yielded to sickness, were then heavy and dull. And as nigh death in their look as ever he saw any.[5]

Charles V, despite his maladies, was an effective ruler, but he became quite depressed when his wife died. His marriage to Isabella was a happy one, as they were both devoted to one another. Sadly, during the first trimester of her seventh pregnancy, Isabella came down with a fever that caused her to miscarry. Infection had taken over, and her health declined quickly. She died two weeks after her stillborn son, in May of 1539. Charles was utterly devastated and shut himself away in a monastery for two months.

The emperor's reaction to his wife's passing is reminiscent of his mother. It seemed he never quite recovered after his wife's death, in much the same way Juana was never the same after the death of Charles's father. For the rest of his life, to show his eternal mourning for her soul, he dressed in black and never remarried, which was almost unheard of for royalty. He commissioned several portraits of Isabella to be painted and kept these portraits with him wherever he travelled.

Perhaps it was the death of his wife that caused him to abdicate the throne at age 58, as he had simply lost interest in ruling. In September of 1558, Charles died due to malarial fever and complications from his lifelong gout.

With the death of Charles V, the Habsburg dynasty would split in two. The rule over Spain went to Charles's son, Philip II, and the Holy Roman Empire went to his brother, Ferdinand I. And intermarriage between the two sides of the family would continue.

If we follow the Spanish line of the Habsburgs, we learn that Philip II would inherit Portugal and Spain. Philip married four times in his life, and all four wives were also relatives, thus thickening the spider's web of genetic complications for the dynasty.

Philip's first marriage was to Maria Manuela, Princess of Portugal (1527–1545), in November 1543. Philip and Maria were double first cousins, as she was the daughter of Philip's maternal uncle and his paternal aunt. Maria and Philip shared all four of their grandparents. Maria gave birth to a son in 1545, but she died a few days later from a haemorrhage.

Their son, Carlos, Prince of Asturias (1545–1568), was not a healthy child. He had a physical deformity, with one leg being shorter than the other, and his shoulders were of a different height. He also had a speech impediment and was plagued by bouts of fever. At the age of 17, after a fall resulted in brain injury, he was given trepanation surgery. A hole was drilled into his skull to release fluid that may have been putting pressure on his brain. While he was lucky to have even survived the operation, he ended up losing his sight for a short time afterwards.

Aside from his disturbing appearance, Carlos also had a very violent temper and was said to have aggressive behaviour toward those around him. He was cruel to animals and derived enjoyment from riding his horses to the point where they would die from exhaustion. These actions seemed to be exacerbated by his abuse of alcohol.

Carlos also had a high-pitched voice, suggesting that the prince had a low level of testosterone. In 1567, he was subjected to a course of remedies to prove or disprove his ability to father a child, to no avail.

The prince died in confinement at age 23. He was rumoured to have exhibited the same gluttonous attitude towards food as his grandfather, Charles. He liked to gorge himself on highly spiced foods and ended up drinking almost ten litres of water in one sitting to quench his thirst from the spices. He died of colic after that incident.

As the only son of Philip II, Carlos was the sole hope for the Habsburg Dynasty for quite some time and after his death, Philip was left without an heir.

Philips's second marriage, in 1554, was to his first cousin once removed, Mary Tudor, queen of England. The couple had no children, and Mary died in 1558.

His third marriage was to Elizabeth of Valois (1545–1568), his third cousin. During the nine years of their marriage, the couple conceived five daughters and one son, but only two of the girls would survive. A son was born stillborn in 1560, twin daughters were miscarried in 1564, and a child born in 1568 died shortly after birth. Elizabeth died only a few hours after the death of their last child.

His fourth wife, Anna of Austria (1549–1580), whom he married in 1570, produced five children. But only one son, Philip III, would live past the age of seven, and Anna died several months after the birth of a daughter in 1580.

The practice of intermarriage would continue with Philip III (1578–1621), who inherited the throne from his father. Philip, who was known for being a less-than-effective and miserable person, married his second cousin, Margaret of Austria (1584–1611). The couple

144

had five children, who all lived to adulthood. Philip's heir, Philip IV (1605–1655), assumed the throne at the age of 16.

Philip IV, born at the Royal Palace of Valladolid, was married to 13-year-old Elisabeth of France (1602–1644) when he was only 10 years old. It is rumoured that Philip fathered over thirty children through his many mistresses. However, out of his ten children with Elisabeth, only two would survive past infancy.

Their only son and heir apparent, Balthasar Charles (1629–1646), was betrothed to his first cousin, Mariana of Austria (1634–1696). However, Charles died from smallpox at the age of 16. His death was quick, which may have been due to his compromised immune system. While Philip was devastated by the death of his son, it didn't stop him from marrying his fiancé Mariana in 1649 – who was also Philip's niece. Philip was 44 and Mariana was just 14.

Philip's marriage to Mariana was guided by his desire to strengthen the relationship with the Austrian Habsburgs. All eight of the couple's grandparents descended from Juana the Mad and Philip I. The couple had two daughters at the beginning of their marriage, with only one surviving to adulthood. Their first son, Philip Prospero (1657–1661), only lived to the age of three. He was a sickly child with a weakened immune system and epilepsy, which caused his death.

Philip and Mariana were convinced that the death of their children was a punishment from God and had no understanding that the family's incessant inbreeding likely caused it. After losing another son in childhood, Mariana finally gave birth to a surviving son, who would become King Charles II of Spain (1661–1700), the most inbred monarch to rule Europe.

On 6 November 1661, Mariana began to feel the symptoms of labour and made her way to the Tower Chamber, which had been prepared for her delivery, with an abundance of sacred relics placed around the room. A team of medical experts was with her, consisting of the royal obstetrician with forty years of experience, the royal midwife, Ines Ayala (1590–1663), who had twenty-five years of experience assisting with royal births, and five other learned doctors.

The king, along with the royal court, knew that Spain's future was entirely dependent on the birth of a son. Doctors had a lot of concern, given the queen's unfortunate history with childbirth, which had resulted in several stillborn children. Mariana also had a history of difficult pregnancies and births, and during the pregnancy of her third child, she suffered several seizures, which almost caused her death. However, her delivery of Charles II was relatively easy, and all were overjoyed at the birth of a son.

The official gazette published that the newborn was: 'Most beautiful in features, with a large head and dark skin and somewhat plump.'

But in the words of the French Ambassador to be, Charles was described as: 'quite weak; he shows signs of degeneration: he has gumboils on his cheeks, his head is full of scabs, and his neck oozes.'

Court astrologers promised a long and happy life for Charles.

Of the fifty-six ancestors of the new heir's mother, forty-eight of them were also the ancestors of his father. The Habsburgs had long felt that their intermarriages were the key to political greatness; in truth, they were also the gateway to a biological hell. The country of Spain was also in a tough spot socially during the time of Charles's birth. Famine, depleted armies, bad harvests, and disease plagued the country.

As a small child, Charles was said to be ugly, and with a deformity to his right ear which was kept covered by his bonnet. There were even rumours that speculated whether or not Charles had recognisable sex organs. But outside the palace doors, the public image of the new king was one of pure fantasy. Because there was a strong belief in the divinity of kings in Spain, Charles was seen as a supreme being. In truth, he had inherited a sacred duty that he would never be able to fulfil.

Immediately following his birth, Dr Bravo and other court doctors were busy organising his milk supply, as plenty of wet nurses were to be considered. Being the wet nurse for a prince was a considerable responsibility, and so the chosen woman had to meet strict regulations. She must be older than 20 but younger than 40, with two or three children of her own. She must be healthy with good daily habits and of a good size. Her breasts must be of ample supply, and she must be cheerful, chaste, sober and without any fits of melancholy. Wet nurses to royalty were not to be of any Jewish or Moorish descent, and a great deal of investigation was done into the heritage of all those considered for this important task. While there was one chosen wet nurse, several others were always waiting to take over should the need arise. Until the age of 4, Charles was breastfed by four different capable wet nurses. By this time, his nursing would cease as it was not considered suitable for a monarch to be breastfed.

Charles's older sister, Maria Theresa, was married to King Louis XIV of France, and so Charles's birth posed a possible threat to Louis, who took great curiosity in the boy. He sent French dignitaries to find out more about him – and from what the dignitaries saw, a rumour was soon started that Charles may not be a boy: 'He appears very feeble, he has a rash on both cheeks, his head is covered in scales and there is a matter protruding from his right ear though it was mostly covered by a bonnet.'[6]

Louis doubted the Spanish heir would live very long, and this notion increased his desire to conquer Spain. From what he understood, Charles was weak and sickly as a child, with frequent diarrhoea and colds. His muscles were not adequately developing, which presented a noticeable delay in his motor development.

In 1665, King Philip became ill and died, leaving the Spanish kingdom to a four-year-old who was being weaned from breast milk, could not yet walk, and had to be carried everywhere by his nurses. Because Charles was just four years old when he was crowned, his regency was administered by his mother, and his father's will instructed him to be declared legal to rule at age 14.

French diplomats who came to offer their condolences on the death of Philip observed Charles's physical struggles.

> The king of Spain supported himself on his feet, propped against the knees of his nurse who held him by the strings of his dress. He covered his head with an English-style

bonnet, which he had not the energy to raise. He seems extremely weak, with pale cheeks and a very open mouth. According to the opinion of his doctors, it is due to some gastric upset. They do not foretell a long life for him.[7]

Aside from a childhood filled with a plethora of viruses, such as measles, chickenpox, rubella and smallpox, Charles was still walking with assistance at age 6. His doctors were continuously mystified that he remained alive. His tongue was so huge, and his jaw so misaligned that he didn't speak until the age of 8, although his speech was not understood. He also had problems chewing his food and often swallowed it whole, which caused him to vomit it back up.

Young Charles also suffered from epileptic seizures that began in his early teens. Along with this, his intellectual development was very poor. He was known for his unpredictable tantrums and an insatiable addiction to chocolate. His speech only became clearly understood at the age of 10. Because it was assumed he would die at a young age due to his poor health, the young king's education was neglected. No one took any time to prepare him for the tasks of government that a king would encounter, and he never learned to write correctly. His tutors struggled to teach him to read and write, and Charles often threw tantrums.

When he was 14, his mother, the queen regent, appointed Fernando de Valenzuela (1636–1692), a court loyalist, to befriend Charles. Under his tutelage, Charles took a keen interest in hunting, though he would never excel at it.

On 6 November 1675, his mother's regency ended as Charles was now of age to officially become king. Spain was now led by a monarch who was sickly, poorly educated, possessed no physical or mental stamina, and was innocent of all worldly knowledge, politics, or diplomacy. When Charles finally did take the throne, plans were immediately put in place for a successor.

Nonetheless, the hope for an heir was the number one goal for any king and queen, and it was decided that Charles should marry within a few years. He was brought up believing that he would marry an

Austrian Princess as this would maintain the family's close genetic bond. It was hoped that he would marry a daughter of his sisters, but no eligible girls were born.

France and Spain's tensions seemed to be at a standstill at the time, and King Louis made a generous offering. Marie Luisa de Orleans (1662–1689), his brother's daughter, would make the perfect bride. The Spanish ambassador promised that she was: 'of remarkable artistry and physique and well modelled with dark hair and eyes and most to the point, apt for immediate fertilisation'.[8]

Marie Louise was indeed very beautiful with a frivolous temperament. She excelled as a horsewoman and was a talented dancer. She wasn't overly intellectual and had little interest in politics but came from a long line of fertile women. In the eyes of the Spanish Court, she was great wife material.

Chances are, her Uncle Louis probably kept her in the dark about the appearance of her soon-to-be husband. The French king was well aware of the deformity of Charles's jaw and the fact that he could hardly swallow his food. He also knew of his reoccurring fevers and rashes and told one of his court ambassadors.

> The prince had passed his life in profound ignorance. Never have they explained to him his own interests and the unique maxim in which they have endeavoured to instruct him the extreme aversion to France. His own inclination has kept him from business and timidly makes him hate the world. His temperament is impulsive, choleric and induces in his extreme melancholy. The sadness which possesses his spirit had the effect of stimulating the infirmities which afflict him.[9]

In November of 1679, at the age of 18, Charles II married Maria Luisa, and one year later, she was still not pregnant. While Charles fell in love immediately, Maria could hardly look at her new husband. Meanwhile, all of Spain waited with bated breath for an heir.

Despite his usual weaknesses, there was one event that seemed to please King Charles very much. The auto-da-fé, on 30 June 1680, proved to be a morbid affair that delighted the king. The Spanish ritual of public punishment was repeatedly carried out between the fifteenth and nineteenth centuries. Heretics and apostates were sentenced to death, tortured, and, in most cases, burned alive.

The summer heat was already overbearing by 8 am that day, but King Charles and his queen would sit for hours during the ordeal. Nineteen people were to be burned by the end of the day. Those who were shown mercy were strangled first. Charles believed that all were condemned according to God's will. During the day, the king appeared almost inebriated by watching the ordeals and in fact, had shown a fondness for the Inquisition since he was four years old and hinted more than once to his mother that he would love to watch the executions.

The auto-da-fé was an event celebrated in splendour and took more than a month to prepare, as people would be gathered in the streets and watching from their windows. The day's events took place in the theatre in the Plaza Mayor, where the king and queen could watch the entire thing. When they arrived, they took their seats on the 29th balcony and stayed there until evening. Everyone was amazed at how composed the king was. He stayed on his balcony, only leaving to go to the bathroom or grab a small bite to eat.

How could an ill, deformed 18-year-old sit in layers of thick clothing for almost fourteen hours? Some say that Charles was cast into a hypnotic trance by the end of the day, perhaps in some half-conscious state induced by exhaustion and fear. Or did he truly enjoy watching people be tortured in the name of God?

Charles and Maria Louisa seemed to settle in rather well for the first few years of their marriage. She certainly enjoyed the new wardrobe and rich food at court. And together, she and Charles enjoyed music and hunting. However, it is likely that the marriage was never properly consummated.

Things eventually began to sour between the couple. Maria Lousia was comforted by the company of several animals at court – including her parrot, which spoke French. This irritated many at court, and in turn, Charles had all her pet parrots killed. Charles began to send her French servants away and decided he would rather hunt alone. He often retired to his bed chamber without saying a word to his queen, not so much as a goodnight, and was slowly seeming to hate anything and everything French. He continuously insulted France in front of her, but she was quick to insult Spain in retaliation.

The royal couple argued so much that people began to worry whether they could tolerate each other long enough to conceive an heir. Charles certainly didn't hide the fact that he thought his wife to be beautiful, nor did he hide his enthusiasm for being physical. The king seemed to find an abnormal amount of time self-stimulating.[10] Biological assumptions could be made today that he suffered from psycho-sexual impotence, or problems getting an erection. He may have also been plagued with premature ejaculation, and it's entirely possible that he was unable to achieve penetration. Neither the king nor queen had any prior knowledge of sexual intercourse, how to handle it, and perhaps, what it even was.

There is a good chance that Charles felt overly anxious as well because he constantly lived with the pressure of knowing it was up to him to carry on the family lineage. But the queen likely thought she was to blame for not getting pregnant because history continuously records that if a couple was infertile, it was the fault of the woman. However, it was also expected that a husband should have some idea of what he should be doing in the marriage bed, but because Charles was so chaste, it's possible he was quite clueless about how to conduct himself.[11]

The couple's inability to conceive an heir only caused them to get on each other's nerves more, and by this time, the Spanish Court had serious disdain for their French queen. When her uncle, Louis XIV, sent several ambassadors to find out what was going on in the marriage bed, we can assume he was not surprised. After all,

Louis himself was known to be quite fond of the company of women and certainly understood the actions that led to pregnancy.

A young diplomat named Rebenac wrote of his accounts on 23 December 1688:

> Finally, Sire, she once told me that she was anxious to confide in me something she never wanted to tell anyone. Namely that she was not really a virgin any longer but that, as far as she could figure things out, she believed she could never have children. Her modesty prevented her from explaining any more fully, and my respect prevented me from asking questions. But I gathered from what she said that there was a natural disability, which was attributed to too much vivacity on the king's part, and finally, Sire, that the action, as the doctor's call, was not perfect.[12]

Rebenac also told King Louis about the Spanish king's undergarments:

> I have found the secret of how to get hold of some of the king's drawers because not to forget any details. He does not wear his shirts longer than to his waist and wears them with a very thick towel which can rub him hard. I have had them examined by two surgeons. One believed that generations may follow, but the other assures me, no.[13]

Rebenac also said that he heard rumours that king and queen were bewitched. He said there was a way to break that spell, but both had to lay totally naked while monks performed an exorcist over them. However, the Catholic Church would never approve of such indecency.

The hatred for Maria Lousia by the Spanish deepened, and they saw her as a failure and a trickster. They were convinced she was sent from Louis to prevent a Spanish heir, but Charles refused to believe his queen was capable of such treachery.

On 8 February 1689, the queen was about to go horseback riding with friends when she stumbled while attempting to mount her horse. She was thrown to the ground and begged her ladies not to speak of the embarrassing incident. That evening she went to bed early after a light meal.

The following day, she complained of a fever and feared she had been poisoned. Her complaints of nausea, stomach pain and diarrhoea continued, and doctors diagnosed her with cholera and an unhealthy diet.

By 11 February, things had worsened for the queen. Her heart began to fail, and she was given an emulsion of opium, salt, and egg yolks. Plasters were applied, along with cupping of the stomach. In the early hours of 12 February, Maria Louisa died. Doctors blamed her poor diet and the cholera, but others questioned whether she had been poisoned. Medical reports on her autopsy gave no answers, as poisoning and bacteria appear much the same way in the gut. During the seventeenth century, it was not rare to consider poisoning as the cause of death. We know today that Maria Luisa died from acute appendicitis, and her autopsy revealed a fully intact and unremarkable uterus. Still, she was considered a disgrace to the royal family because she did not give birth to an heir. Many saw her as an obstacle that was out of the way, so the court could focus on getting a proper heir from their king. Louis XIV was not concerned with the possibility of an heir and saw no threat in a new marriage for Charles, as he believed he was just too unhealthy to reproduce.

Charles was still in constant poor health at the age of 28. He was always weak and tired and suffered frequent gastrointestinal problems, which were made worse by his obsession with sugary food and inability to chew his food. He showed signs of distress at his wife's death for a little over a week, but he appeared to have gotten over it quickly. He seemed to want to be left alone. He said he never wanted to marry again as it was too overwhelming. He stated that he believed the death of his wife and their childless marriage was God's punishment.

Nevertheless, Chares II was still seen as the one true hope to carry on the Habsburg dynasty, and only ten days after his wife died, he was pressured by his council to remarry and produce an heir. It was decided on Maria Anna of Neuburg (1667–1740). She was nine of twenty-two siblings, so clearly, fertility was not a problem, and it was imperative that not even one hour be wasted on getting her to court. On 24 August, the couple were married by proxy, and ten days later, Maria Anna began her treacherous journey to Spain.

She travelled down the Danube to Dusseldorf, where she was delayed until 6 November before continuing down the Rhine. Maria was kept well nourished on her trip with a diet including smoked ham and butter, but it was growing colder by the day, and the Rhine was beginning to ice over. On 24 December, she was transferred to an English fleet as they had agreed to assist in transporting her to Spain. However, the river was so frozen that a group of horses had to pull the ship through the chunks of ice.

On 28 January, Maria was transferred to a much more pleasurable vessel where she was given her own cabin with comfortable chairs and warm blankets. But she was so seasick that she went straight to bed. She was still onboard the ship on 4 March – a year since it was stated at the Spanish Court that not even one hour could be wasted on getting her to Spain. Maria's doctor and her barber surgeon were also seasick, along with two of her ladies. On 26 March, a huge windstorm blew their ship off course and ripped two of its sails off.

Finally, on 4 May 1690, the couple met in person, and the marriage was officially confirmed. While all her sisters had no trouble getting pregnant, the same could not be said for Maria. Children would never be created in the marriage bed of Charles and Maria. However, the new queen also saw her marriage to Charles as a way to give her small German family more credibility.

Not surprisingly, conversations were overheard at court of the queen saying that Charles's sexual behaviour was disappointing, and she considered that he might be bewitched. She wrote to her father that next month after her marriage to Charles about how miserable she was in Spain. By October of that year, her health began to decline with depression, headaches, and indigestion. She was in considerable pain and resigned herself to death. But surprisingly, the queen began to recover, which was credited to Spain's superior medical care: 'Spanish treatment is unlike the Germans. Here the doctors give the patient a drink of iced water before and after the purge instead of a hot liquid.'[14]

Once Maria Anna recovered, all concentration was put on helping her to conceive. This was also something Spanish and German doctors could not agree on. The Spanish thought she should drink the water of Puertollano, which was said to help with fertility. But her German doctor disagreed and suggested a visit to Valladolid: 'It is essential to correct, by a change of air, the disequilibrium between their majesties temperament for otherwise, they will never have heirs.'[15]

While she was eventually given the water treatment, we must question whether nor not either of these doctors really believed that the problem with infertility lay with the queen.

Along with her entourage, Maria Anna began to find ways to smuggle money, furniture, jewels, and tapestries from the royal palaces to Germany. It is also suspected that she put her energy into coaxing Charles to put her family in his will, but he was also swayed by his mother not to do so. Trying to keep both women happy often sent him into a rage. Maria often threatened Charles, saying she would starve herself if he didn't include her family in the will.

Maria Anna probably understood that the problem with conceiving an heir lay with Charles, as she was less naïve than his former queen. She may have been told formally not to expect much in the procreation department. She seemed to suffer times of emotional stress over having to be intimate with the king. She was said to have suffered epilepsy several times while in the marriage bed, though it never seemed to plague her when she slept alone.

The relationship between the queen and the queen mother became toxic. The queen mother tried to convince her son to be rid of the queen as she was sterile and useless. But for the most part, he refused to listen to her.

* * * *

During the seventeenth century in Madrid, the month of March was one devoted to getting rid of all the evil humours that had built up during the winter – purging and bloodletting were quite popular during this month. In March of 1696, the queen's mother disclosed to her doctors that she had a lump in her breast that had grown to the size of a pomegranate. Of course, the treatment was to bleed her once again. The queen mother's doctors believed that a cancer plagued her. An operation was not an option; instead, they believed that weakening her and using evacuation methods was the answer. Doctors made her vomit with their medications, and her fevers continued to rise, and they inevitably knew their methods were useless.

Jesuits from the Imperial Society of Madrid were convinced her cancer was a pagan carcinoma: masses were said in her honour, and holy relics were brought to her bedside. Nonetheless, she died on 16 May 1696. There are not a lot of records telling us how Charles reacted to the death of his mother, and at the time, he was very ill himself.

Hopes were still high at court that Queen Maria Anna was able to get pregnant, and things such as a bout of nausea or feeling sad, gave everyone hope that she was with child.

In June of that year, her physician wrote to her brother in Germany about the hopes of a pregnancy: 'She is shivering throughout her body, sick with headache, having vertigo and frequent nausea. She is vomiting with a weak pulse and aversion to food.'[16]

However, her brother was the wiser and knew she was not pregnant and must have been suffering from an illness of sorts. He was sure this was all just a result of her misery at the Spanish Court.

By March of 1698, the health of King Charles was in decline. It was written that he was very weak and could hardly lift his head to eat. He was so miserable that nothing could make him smile. He also began to realise that the reason Spain had no heir was no fault of his queen. It was because of him.

The king was convinced that a spell had been cast against him, which prevented him from being able to procreate. While he understood that he could not father children, he still believed it was God's will rather than a physical disorder. In the seventeenth century, impotence was considered to be the result of one of two things: you either suffered from natural frigidity, or you were impotent by witchcraft. Charles was easily convinced that he was bewitched as he had always been obsessed with the thought of the devil working evil in his life.

Complementum Artis Exorcisiacae by Zacharius Vicecomite told Charles all he needed to know about being bewitched:

> Bewitched people crave the worse kinds of food and are vexed by solid food. They cannot retain the food they take and are molested by continuous vomiting. Others have always had indigestion and feel a heavy weight on their stomach. Some feel a bolus frequency ascending from the stomach to the throat, which they seem to vomit. And nevertheless, it seconds to its original position. With others, there is a gnawing at the mouth of the belly. Others feel a frequent throbbing in their neck, often at the same hour of each day. With others, there is a continuous unnatural pain in the head and brain with which they seem to be weighed down, shattered and transfixed. The heart of a bewitched person is afflicted in such a way that he feels torn by dogs or serpents or pieced by nails of steel or suffocated. With some, the viscera are tortured, and the stomach is intensely and frequently inflated. Many bewitched people are loaded down by a melancholic humour which makes some so infirm that

they die not willing to speak of hold converse with men.
A very notable sign of bewitchment is when medicines
administered do not help the sufferers.[17]

After reading this, it is easy to understand how Charles could not
have seen himself in the writing. But he also wondered if he was
not bewitched, he was surely possessed, as that was the only other
explanation.

In the same book, Vicecomite writes about possession:

> Often possessed people have swollen and blackened
> tongues protruding from their mouths in an unnatural
> manner or their throat is inflated or constricted. They yell
> without knowing why. They reply angrily when asked
> questions. Even when forced to talk, they do not want
> to. They clench their teeth and refuse to eat. They pursue
> men with hatred. They talk much with little meaning.
> They are oppressed with heavy stupor. They remain
> senseless from time to time. They persecute themselves,
> tearing their clothes and their hair. They have terrible,
> horrible eyes. They are afflicted with sudden terrors that
> quickly disappear. They imitate the sounds of various
> animals, the roaring of lions, the bleating of sheep, and
> the lowering of oxen. The barking of dogs, grunting of
> pigs, and the like. They grind their teeth and foam at the
> mouth and show other similarities to a mad dog. Fire
> carries through their bodies or an icy vapour. They feel as
> if ants are moving through their bodies, or frogs jumping
> or vipers and serpents or fish swimming, flies flying, and
> the like. They yell and hear various things contrary to
> matter.[18]

While it may seem ridiculous today, much of this described Charles
perfectly. All the horrible sensations and unnatural gestures he

experienced in his life were laid out before him. It's hard not to sympathise with him because he knew no better and to think that you may be housing a demon of some sort must have been terrifying for the king. Charles's only hope at the time was to pray that he was only bewitched and not fully possessed.

Two years prior, Charles already had suspicions and sent for the Inquisitor General. While he seriously considered that Charles might be bewitched, that was as far as it was taken.

In 1698, an investigation into the matter was launched. Those looking into the problem concluded that Charles had indeed been the victim of a spell. They stated that on 3 April 1675, he was given a cup of chocolate that held the dissolved brains of an executed man to curse the government. Dissolved entrails and kidneys were also included, which compromised his health and made him unable to father children.

Father Froylan, one of the king's later confessors, was still not totally convinced and was intent on finding out why Charles was impotent. Was it natural, or was he truly bewitched? Would he need an exorcism? Talks of such a thing were bold on Father Froylan's behalf, and he knew it was not something the Catholic Church took lightly. A priest performing an exorcism put himself at great risk as he would be vulnerable to the devil's tactics.

The Inquisitor General and Father Froylan wanted an exorcism, but Bishop Tomás Reluz, Bishop of Oviedo (1636–1709), wanted nothing to do with it. He thought the business about the king being bewitched was nonsense. But if the exorcism were to be carried out, Father Antonio Arquelles would conduct it. However, he was uncertain about going against the bishop and wanted specific instructions from the Inquisitor General in writing. Father Antonio had experience with the ritual and understood it was not to be taken lightly.

Father Antonio first suggested that the king be given a fast, a ½ pint of olive oil which had been duly blessed according to the exorcism ritual. He must eat slowly, and everything he ate or drank should be blessed. There was no time to waste. Exorcisms were not foreign to the king as he had been put through a series of exorcisms during his life and made to drink potions which only made him worse. Holy relics were also brought to the king along with the bones of his deceased father in the hopes that the evils in his body would leave.

Both Charles and his queen were also given other treatments approved by the church, such as bleeding, purging and enemas. In December 1698, a Jeronite Friar exorcised the queen to make her fertile, assuming the devil had deemed her infertile. The exorcism ritual was not nearly as unpleasant as the remedies or treatments prescribed by seventeenth-century doctors.

By the summer of the next year, the king's health took a turn for the worse. He was so weak that he was unable to stay on his feet for more than an hour. His tongue had swollen to the point where he was unable to speak. His daily living consisted of exhaustion, seizures, fever, and diarrhoea.

> His Catholic Majesty grows every day sensibly worse and worse. Thursday, they made him walk in the public procession of Corpus, which was much shortened for his sake. However, he performed so feebly that all who saw him said he could not make one straight step but staggered all the way. Nor could it otherwise be expected after he had had two falls a day before walking in his own lodgings when his legs doubled under him from mere weakness. In one of them, he hurt one eye, which appeared to be much swelled black and blue in the procession, and the other being quite sunk into his head. The nerves, they say, being contracted by is paralytic distemper. Yet it was thought fit to have him make this sad figure in public only to have it put into the gazette how strong and vigorous he was.[19]

So once again, we see evidence of the truth and the falsities that were told by the Gazette, which blindly led the public to believe their king was well.

That summer proved to be another of the hottest in Madrid, but the king was so cold and shivering that he had to have several blankets placed over him.

By March 1700, all hope that Charles Habsburg would produce an heir to secure the family dynasty was lost. Thoughts were turned to whether the House of Bourbon or the House of Habsburg should reign when the succession was brought up. All talk of the bewitched king was put aside.

On 6 June, Charles ordered the Council of State to meet but refused to attend as he wanted no influence over their discussions. One thought was that the king of France's grandson would inherit the Spanish throne but that the two kingdoms must never merge. This idea left Louis XIV with a complicated diplomacy.

If Charles left the empire to Austria, the rest of Europe may rise up against it. But if he left it to France, it was uncertain what would arise. Finally, Charles decided that the Duke of Anjou, the second son of the dauphin should be his heir.

During the last days of King Charles II, the queen fed him some tapioca starch called 'milk of pearls' by hand. He soon went completely deaf. To prevent vertigo, his doctors put Spanish flies on his feet and freshly killed pigeons on his head. During the evening of 29 June, they tried to keep him warm by putting freshly killed animal entrails on his stomach. He soon lost all ability to speak and slipped into a coma. Charles II died at 2.49 pm on 1 November 1700.

The autopsy of the king revealed that his heart was very small, about the size of a nut. There were stone in his liver, his kidneys were filled with water and his intestines were putrid. He also had a single black testicle and a head full of water.

His death was assumed to have been caused by witchcraft. A medical diagnosis today would conclude that he suffered from posterior hypospadias monorchism, a problem in the development of the penis in which the urethra does not open from the head of the penis. He most likely suffered from an atrophic testicle and multiple genitalia. The stones found were likely kidney stones and infections.

Medical historians believe that Charles suffered from a plethora of genetic diseases, including distal renal tubular acidosis, pituitary hormone deficiency, Klinefelter Syndrome, Fragile X Syndrome, acromegaly, and hydrocephalus. The king's late growth and compromised mental development, as well as his frequent vomiting and epileptic seizures, particularly speak to hydrocephalus.

His urological problems were most likely attributed to Klinefelter Syndrome, which included small testicles and a short penis. Klinefelter Syndrome is a genetic condition affecting boys, who are born with an extra copy of the X chromosome, and it usually isn't diagnosed until adulthood. It usually affects testicular growth, resulting in a lower production of testosterone. Most men diagnosed with Klinefelter syndrome produce little, if any, sperm, which of course, would be the primary reason why neither of Charles's wives became pregnant.

Fragile X Syndrome is another genetic condition that is much more severe in males. There is a delay of speech and language that is usually evident by the age of 2, and most have moderate intellect. Children with the disorder also exhibit hyperactivity and impulsive actions, which may have been manifested in the tantrums Charles would throw. The disorder also increases the chance of seizures. The physical features of one with Fragile X Syndrome include a long and narrow face, which Charles had. Large ears and a prominent jaw, as well as flat feet, are also characteristics of Fragile X.

If Charles suffered from acromegaly, it would explain the large bone structure found in his feet and hands as well as his face.

As mentioned above, hydrocephalus could have contributed to many of the king's ailments. With the excessive build up of fluid in the brain, much pressure is put on the structures and internal workings of the organ. Too much cerebrospinal fluid can not only damage brain tissue but cause a variety of problems.

Hydrocephalus causes an unusually large head and bulging fontanel, which could explain why the fontanels on his head took so long to close. The king's consistent vomiting and poor eating, as well as his lethargy, along with his inability to walk properly, could also be attributed to hydrocephalus.

However, aside from all the other disorders that Charles II suffered, he was most known for mandibular prognathism, or the Habsburg Jaw. The word prognathism comes from the Greek word for forward, which is appropriate, given the disorder produces a jaw that protrudes forward, often resulting in another condition called malocclusion, where the top and lower teeth do not align properly.

Charles was the last of the male line of the Spanish Habsburg, ending the centuries-long dynasty. While the throne should have gone to the heir of his oldest sister, Maria Theresa (1638–1683), Charles wrote in his will that it should instead go to Philip, Duke of Anjou (1683–1746), the grandson of King Louis XIV of France. This resulted in the War of Spanish Succession (1701–174), which lasted 13 years. When it was announced that France and Spain were to unite, a backlash from England, Holland, Prussia, and Austria ensued, as it was a move that jeopardised the balance of power in Europe. Nonetheless, Louis and Maria Theresa's grandson, who became Philip V, would take the throne, establishing Bourbon rule over Spain.

* * * *

The Habsburgs, like many of the royal families of Europe, were intent on maintaining social order by ensuring that royals and nobles always sat at the top of the feudal ladder. Aside from this, politics were incredibly important, which was why so many peace treaties were sealed with a marriage. Young brides were forever being sent to live with their new husbands to keep nations from going to war. Because the Habsburgs had two branches, this only made the family inbreeding so much worse. The Habsburgs were often short of male heirs (due to their inbreeding), so daughters of the Holy Roman Empire were usually married to the Spanish Habsburgs to ensure that the next rule would be mostly Habsburg.

The Austrian line of the Habsburgs also dates to Rudolph I, who took control of the Grand Duchy of Austria in 1278. Austria was part of the Holy Roman Empire, and in 1437, Fredrick III (1415–1493) took it over when the predecessor died without an heir. Fredrick was the fourth king and the first emperor of the House of Habsburg.

Frederick married Eleanor of Portugal (1434–1467), and their son, Maximillian I, married Mary Duchess of Burgundy (1457–1482). But when Mary died at the age of 25 after falling from her horse, France went to war with the Holy Roman Empire over her inheritance. Burgundy went to France while the Netherlands went to Maximillian, and the couple's son, Philip the Handsome married Juana the Mad, making him the first Habsburg to rule Spain.

As we know, the son of Philip and Juana, Charles V, would inherit the Holy Roman Empire from his grandfather. We know that Maximillian had become very depressed in his fifties and began to have his coffin brought with him wherever he went. When he died at 59, he had left instructions on how his corpse should be handled. He wished for his hair to be cut off and his teeth to be knocked out, his body whipped and covered in lime and ash. We can assume that Maximillian may have suffered from some form of mental illness, and while it may not have been from inbreeding, the trait was passed down to his children and grandchildren.

When Charles V died, the Holy Roman Empire went to his younger brother, Ferdinand I, thus ensuring the long dispute over whether the Habsburgs would be divided in two. Eventually, Ferdinand married Anne of Bohemia and Hungary (1503–1547). Anne was unrelated to any Habsburg, so their genetics were not compromised. The couple went on to have fifteen children.

The couple's son, Maximillian II (1527–1576) inherited the Holy Roman Empire, only to reintroduce the inbred traits inherited from his father. He also married his cousin, the daughter of Charles V, Maria of Austria (1528–1603). Out of their sixteen children, eight reached adulthood. Maximillian was plagued by ill health for most of his life, and at the age of 49 he died of heart failure.

The couple's eldest daughter, Anna of Austria, married her Spanish uncle, Philip II of Spain, while their eldest son, Rudolph II (1552–1612) became the next Holy Roman Emperor.

Anna and Philip's marriage was a happy and loving one. Anna was adored by her husband, and he took no mistresses during his marriage to her. Anna gave birth to five children, but only one reached adulthood which is easy to understand due to their close kinship.

Anna's brother, Rudolph II, was an unpopular ruler who died without an heir. He never married, though he is reported to have several illegitimate children through mistresses. While we don't know much about the mental health of Rudolph himself, other than he suffered from bouts of melancholy, the mental health of one of his illegitimate children is well documented. His son, Julius (1584–1609), was sent to live at Český Krumlov, a castle that Rudolph owned. It was there that he reportedly abused and murdered a local barber's daughter who had also been living at the castle. He then disfigured her corpse. Rudolph was appalled at his son's behaviour and suggested he be imprisoned for the remainder of his life. But before this could happen, Julius died. He had begun to show signs of schizophrenia, he refused to bathe himself and lived in total filth; his death followed a ruptured ulcer. Is it possible that somewhere in the genetic pool of the Habsburgs, Julius inherited a very severe form of mental illness?

Rudolph II was an ineffective ruler who was more preoccupied with his artwork and other hobbies, and his unpopularity allowed his brother Matthias (1557–1619) to overthrow him. But Matthias proved to be ineffective and died without an heir.

The throne went to his cousin, Ferdinand II (1578–1637), whose parents were uncle and niece. He had several brothers and sisters who died in infancy because of the close relationship of their parents. And yet, Ferdinand would continue the intermarriage trend, marrying his cousin Maria Anna of Bavaria (1574–1616). Out of their seven children, only four would reach adulthood. When Ferdinand died at age 59, his son, Ferdinand III (1608–1657), inherited the throne.

Because the Austrian and Spanish sides of the Habsburgs had the same idea when it came to persecuting Protestants, any family disputes were brought to an end. Ferdinand III married his cousin, Maria Anna of Spain (1606–1646), to keep the peace, and the two went on to have a relatively happy marriage.

Maria Anna died in childbirth and when Ferdinand married for the second and third time, both his wives were also relatives.

When their oldest son died of smallpox at the age of 21, his younger brother Leopold (1640–1705) would continue the family line. Along with having the typical Habsburg jaw, Leopold was pale-faced, short and thin. Historian William Coxe (1748–1828) described him thus: 'His gait was stately, slow and deliberate; his air pensive, his address awkward, his manner uncouth, his disposition cold and phlegmatic.' A Turkish traveller described Leopold as 'a cultivated man of extreme ugliness'.[20]

But despite this, the push was on to secure the Habsburg dynasty once again. Leopold was said to be deeply in love with his niece, Margaret Theresa of Spain (1651–1673), who was also the sister of Charles II. Portraits of her as a young girl showed a lovely and beautiful child whom Leopold was eager to marry. She was only 15 when she came to court to marry him, and he was 26, eleven years her senior. Leopold was not only her maternal uncle but also her paternal cousin.

As soon as they were married, Leopold was intent on getting his new bride into the marriage bed. He was utterly in awe of her and demanded she call him uncle – especially during lovemaking.

Margaret was somewhat healthier than her unfortunate brother, but during their six-year marriage, only one of her children with Leopold survived infancy, but it was a daughter. Three other children were born with deformities, and in between her deliveries, Margaret suffered many devastating miscarriages. Her scapegoat for the lack of surviving children was the Jews, and she ordered Leopold to expel them from Vienna and destroy their synagogues. She was known for being intensely anti-Semitic. Her short but seemingly miserable life ended in her fifth pregnancy at the age of 21.

Although devastated by his wife's death, Leopold soon married again. This time, Leopold moved on to marry his cousin, Claudia Felicitas of Austria (1653–1676). She was a young and vibrant 21-year-old, while Leopold was now in his mid-thirties. Leopold didn't care for his second wife as much as he had for Margaret, but it would not matter in the end. Both couple's children died only a few months after birth, and Claudia succumbed to tuberculosis and died at age 22, leaving Leopold once again without an heir.

After twenty years on the throne Leopold still had no male heir, and other countries saw this as a weakness. Desperate for an heir, Leopold married another cousin, Eleanor Madalena of Nuremberg (1655–1720). Though she was known to be quite brilliant, Eleanor was not considered pretty, nor was she healthy. However, she was known for the fertility in her family. Leopold ordered his personal physician to examine his new bride and concluded that she was 'fresh enough'. Leopold, now 50, was once again marrying a pry 21-year-old. Eleanor proved her fertility, as the couple had ten children, though only five would survive adulthood.

Leopold was so keen on ruling a large territory that he was intent on marrying into the family. Anything else would have been unthinkable. His obsession with producing an heir would put him through three marriages to family members.

Leopold died at the age of 65 and passed the throne onto his son, Joseph I (1678–1711), who married Vilhelmine Lunia of Brunswick (1673–1742) in February 1699. She was not a close relative, but Joseph was already inbred enough. The couple had three children, but their only son died of hydrocephalus before his first birthday. Because of Joseph's desire for mistresses, he caught syphilis, which he likely passed on to his wife, and this rendered her, if not both, sterile.

Prior to this, Leopold had made both Joseph and his brother, Charles (1685–1740), sign the Mutual Pact of Succession. If neither son fathered a male heir, then the throne would be passed to Joseph's daughters before any daughters of Charles. Because Charles was still alive when Joseph died, however, he inherited the throne as Charles VI.

The wife of Charles VI was Christine of Brunswick (1691–1750), who was not a relative, and the couple had three healthy daughters but no sons. Charles tried to secure his eldest daughter as his heir, but his father's ruling stood in the way. Once his brother Joseph died however, Charles was free to do what he wanted, and he ignored the rule of succession and passed the throne on to his eldest daughter, Maria Theresa (1717–1780). This led to the War of Austrian Succession (1740–1748) when France, Prussia and Bavaria saw this as the perfect opportunity to challenge the great Habsburg power.

Maria Amalia (1701–1756), the youngest daughter of Joseph I, and her husband, Charles VII of Idlesbach (1697–1745), rejected that Charles VI's decision to ignore the rule of succession. As the son-in-law of Joseph I, Charles VII claimed the German territories of the Habsburgs after the death of Charles VI. Charles VII did become Holy Roman Empire for three brief years, temporarily interrupting Habsburg rule, but he died at the age of 48.

Marie Theresa took back her throne and married her second cousin, Francis I (1708–1765). Together, they ruled as co-monarchs. However, it was Marie who was ultimately the decision-maker, as she was an excellent ruler. Together the couple had 16 children, three of who died in infancy. Three also died of smallpox in their teens, most likely from their weakened immune systems due to family inbreeding.

Marie's children, like most royal children, were used as pawns in the game of marriage. Her most well-known daughter was Marie Antionette. Marie Antoinette was just another piece of the political chessboard of the Habsburg dynasty as the family struggled to navigate through the Seven Years' War (1756–1763).

On the evening of 2 November 1755, Marie Antionette was born in Vienna. Though she was primarily placed under the care of her governess, she had a loving relationship with her mother, but at times it was difficult.

Though she was offered private tutoring, by the age of ten, Marie struggled to write correctly in German, French or Italian, and conversations with her were often hard to keep together. However, musically, Marie was talented and had a lovely voice, and she was also described as having good character and a good heart.

History tells us that Marie Antoinette was the epitome of French glamour who adored fine clothes and towering wigs. And while this may have been true, she underwent quite the makeover as a child to suit the political needs of her mother. Though Marie Antoinette was described as very attractive, she still had a protruding lower lip caused by the Habsburg Jaw. Her features were much milder than her relatives and her pout was considered almost adorable.

While her marriage into the French Court was inevitable, when the French envoy, the Duc de Choiseul (1719–1785), first laid eyes on her, he was rather unimpressed. Her manners were poor, her hair unkempt, and her clothes wrinkled.

Her teeth were also crooked; for one in the Bourbon court, this was far from acceptable. Pierre Fauchard (1679–1761), an up-and-coming pioneer, devised a piece shaped like a U that would be fitted into Marie Antoinette's mouth. It was fastened to her teeth by tied strands of gold; over time, it reshaped her dental arch and straightened her crooked teeth. It can be assumed that her crooked teeth were part of the Habsburg jaw disorder, and she suffered through months of dental work that was not done under any anaesthesia.

Maria Theresa ruled for forty years, and when she died at the age of 63, her eldest son, Joseph II (1741–1790), inherited the throne. While Joseph was intelligent, he wasn't kind to his people and soon became unpopular. His first wife, Isabella of Parma (1741–1763), gave birth to three children, but only one would live. Isabella died during childbirth, delivering her fourth child. Joseph was a devoted father to his only daughter, but she died at the age of 7 of a lung infection. Joseph died at the age of 48.

It was during Joseph's reign that his sister, Marie Antionette, married her husband, Louis XVI of France.

Joseph's brother, Leopold II (1747–1792) then became Holy Roman Emperor and married Maria Luisa of Spain (1745–1792), the daughter of Charles III of Spain. The couple had sixteen healthy children.

Their son, Francis II (1768–1835,) would be the last Holy Roman Emperor. Unfortunately for Francis, his father was a staunch disciplinarian and critic. He wrote that Francis was 'stunted in growth, backwards in bodily dexterity and deportment and a spoiled mother's child'.[21] His father filled his life with fear and unpleasantness, keeping young Francis isolated.

Much like his predecessors, Francis II would marry several times. His first wife was Elisabeth of Württemberg (1767–1790), born in modern-day Poland. At the age of 15, she came to Vienna under the direction of Francis's father, and she was educated by nuns and converted to Catholicism to be the perfect future bride to Francis. She delighted her new father-in-law, Emperor Joseph, who found her to be refreshing company, and they enjoyed one another's presence. She saw him as a father or grandfather and would give him much comfort in his last days.

The couple married in early January 1788, and by the end of the following year Elisabeth was pregnant – but in a very grave situation. She received the anointing of the sick for her condition. In February of 1790, she fainted on the night of the 18th before giving birth to a premature baby who would only live sixteen months. Desperate attempts were made to save the life of Elisabeth after a gruelling twenty-four-hour labour, but she sadly died.

Frances II then married his double first cousin, Maria of Naples and Sicily (1772–1807). The marriage between the two was pleasant, even though Francis did not share her personality. He was often depressed and reserved.

Despite sharing four sets of grandparents, the couple had twelve children together, but only seven reached adulthood. In the winter of 1806, while pregnant with their twelfth child, Maria Theresa came down with tuberculosis, which her doctors treated by bleeding her. Not surprisingly, the treatment did not improve her health but instead triggered premature labour. The birth of her daughter, who lived but a few days, caused complications for Maria, and she died a few days later.

Francis II was devastated by his wife's death and had to be forcibly removed from her dead body. He could not face the funeral and instead travelled to Buda. This is not the first time we have heard this tale of a distraught spouse unable to leave the side of their deceased loved one.

Francis would marry two more times, once to Maria Ludwig of Austria (1787–1816) and once to Caroline Charlotte Augusta of Bavaria (1792–1873), neither marriage produced children.

It was during Francis's reign that his aunt, Marie Antoinette, was tried by the Revolutionary Tribunal for treason and found guilty. She was sentenced to be executed in October 1793; a few years later, the French Revolution was in full swing. Francis had never met his aunt and was not ready to compromise his hopes of victory against the French for a woman he did not know.

On the day of her execution, 16 October, she changed into a plain white dress, and her hands were bound behind her back. As she made her way to the guillotine erected in Place de la Revolution, she maintained her composure and dignity, ignoring the insults being slung at her from the crowd. She climbed the stairs to the scaffold with no assistance and, because of her gentle nature, apologised to the executioner when she accidentally stepped on his foot.

She was executed at 12.15 in the afternoon.

Marie Antoinette may have escaped most of the physical and mental abnormalities of the Habsburg genes but she should be remembered – if not for her beauty and kindness. She was also known for being a loving and devoted mother.

* * * *

In 1799, Napoleon (1769–1821) took control of France and called himself emperor. Francis II joined forces with the United Kingdom, Russia, and other nations to revolt against Napoleon, but ended up abdicating the throne, ending the Holy Roman Empire for good.

At this point Napoleon was without an heir; he went on to further strengthen his empire by marrying into one of the leading families in Europe. He married Maria-Louise (1791–1847), the daughter of Francis II and Maria Theresa of Naples and Sicily, securing himself a place in a German Imperial Family.

Francis II died of a sudden fever while in Vienna at age 67. He was given a splendid funeral and buried in the traditional resting place of the Habsburg monarchs.

Francis's son, Ferdinand I (1793–1875), became the next emperor of Austria, the title his father still held at his death. Because both of his parents were related several times over, Ferdinand also suffered from the mutated genes that had plagued the Habsburgs for decades. Ferdinand was born in mid-April 1793 and suffered from several ailments from an early age.

He had severe epilepsy and hydrocephalus, which caused is head to be abnormally large and in a rather alarming disproportion to his small stature. In addition to his physical ailments, Ferdinand also suffered from mental disabilities, which included up to twenty seizures a day.

Ferdinand received little, if any, treatment for his condition, and he was not encouraged in any way as a young boy. He was not even capable of pouring himself a glass of water, climbing the stairs, or opening the door unless he had help. Despite his maladies from inbreeding, Ferdinand is said to have been able to speak five languages and have artistic talents.

In keeping with tradition, as the first-born son he was the heir to the throne and at the age of 25, he made his first appearance as a prince. He was stated as his father's official representative at the time, though most people had very little faith that he was capable of the position.

In 1831, Ferdinand married Maria Anna of Piedmont-Sardinia (1803–1884), who was, not surprisingly, a distant relative. Maria Anna was a meek woman who, at age 27, was said to look old and not to appease the eye. But Maria Anna was also shocked at her future husband's condition when they first met. While trying to consummate the marriage, Ferdinand suffered a terrible epileptic seizure. While the marriage would not produce any heirs, Maria Anna was a kind wife and often referred to herself as her husband's nurse.

An attempt to assassinate Ferdinand was narrowly avoided in 1832. While unharmed physically, he was deeply affected by it emotionally. He was little more than a defacto puppet whose strings were pulled by members of his council.

Revolutions were breaking out in Europe, and Ferdinand was forced to abdicate in favour of his nephew, Franz Joseph I (1830–1916). He later retired to Prague Castle, were he died at the age of 82.

On 18 August 1830, Franz Joseph was born in Schonbrunn Palace in Vienna. Because it was assumed he would inherit the throne from his feeble-minded uncle, Franz was raised as a future monarch would be raised. He was raised under the care of his nanny, Louise von Sturmfeder (1789–1866), where he was dually educated.

By the time he was 16, he was expected to study up to fifty hours a week, focusing on learning several languages, such as Latin, Hungarian, Italian, and Polish. He was also taught history, mathematics, and geography.

Following the abdication of his uncle, Franz Joseph claimed the throne of emperor of Austria on 2 December 1848. No time was wasted in getting the new emperor married so that heirs could be produced as soon as possible. Because his mother wanted to strengthen the relationship between the House of Habsburg and the House of Wittelsbach, from which she descended, she pushed for a marriage to her niece, Helene (1834–1890). But it was Helen's sister, Elisabeth (1837–1898), or Sisi, with whom Franz Joseph found himself in love. The young couple were married in April 1854 in St Augustine's Church, Vienna.

While Franz fell deeper in love with his beautiful young wife, she did not return those feelings. She found herself in conflict with the royal family and never adjusted to life at the Austrian Court. Their first daughter died as an infant, and their only son died in 1889 by way of suicide.

Sisi was a woman who became obsessed with her beauty and spent very little time at court. We will learn more about the empresses of Wittelsbach in the next chapter. When she died in 1898 while on a trip to Vienna, Franz was devastated, claiming, 'you'll never know how important she was to me.'

Because their son would die before his father, the next heir was a nephew – also the result of a marriage of second cousins. Franz Ferdinand (1863–1914) and his wife, Sophie (1868–1914), would be the last generation of Habsburgs to bind themselves together through incestuous marriage.

Perhaps this decision came as a result of the research done by Gregor Mendel, as he had established that hereditary defects had a direct link to inbreeding. Royal families finally took things more seriously and began to look outside the family for a spouse.

Nonetheless, it's possible that Franz Ferdinand still inherited a form of mental illness, as he was known for being angry, violent, and reckless. On June 28, 1914, Franz Ferdinand and his wife were assassinated in Sarajevo as they were perceived as a threat to Serbian independence.

Despite being the last incestuous couple of the Habsburgs, the claws of the family would reach into neighbouring monarchies, and their innate genes would not be far behind.

The modern Habsburg family still survives, without the defective genes of their ancestors. The head of the House of Habsburg-Lorraine today is Karl Von Habsburg, who was born in 1961 and remains in perfect health.

Chapter Eleven

House of Wittelsbach and the Mad Cousins

One of the oldest Catholic dynasties to rule in Europe are the Wittelsbachs. Aside from being famous for being the royal house of Empress Elisabeth of Austria and King Ludwig II of Bavaria (1845–1886), the Wittelsbach empire is also known for its own share of intermarriage. While perhaps not to the extent of the Habsburgs, the Wittelsbach family still managed to produce rulers that suffered the effects of the family's inbreeding.

The House of Wittelsbach ruled in Bavaria from 1180 to 1918. Other branches of the family ruled in Sweden from 1441–1448 and from 1654 to 1720, Hungary in 1305 and Denmark and Norway in 1440. While the Habsburgs were tied with the Holy Roman Emperor in 1742, it was a Wittelsbach who held that title.

Charles VII (1697–1745) was Holy Roman Emperor from 1742 until his death three years later. As a member of the House of Wittelsbach, his reign brought three centuries of Habsburg rule to a halt, even though he was related to the Habsburgs by both blood and marriage.

In the eighteenth century, the ruling of the House of Wittelsbach was split between the Palatinate and Bavaria, which is what eventually brings us to the reigns of Empress Elisabeth and King Ludwig II.

Maximillian Joseph I (1756–1825) was the first Bavarian king. He had several children between his two wives, the first of which was Ludwig I (1786–1868), his heir to the Bavarian throne. Ludwig was king of Bavaria until 1848 when the French Revolution forced him to abdicate in favour of his son Maximillian (1811–1864). Maximillian

Joseph was the grandfather of both Empress Elisabeth and King Ludwig II.

We know that the Wittelsbach family was sporadically inbred, as the son of Maximillian Joseph, Empress Elisabeth's father, married his second cousin, Ludovika of Bavaria (1808–1892).

As mentioned in the previous chapter, the wife of Franz Joseph (House of Habsburg) was Elisabeth of Austria, known as Sisi. Maximillian was delighted at the birth of his daughter, and as it was Christmas Eve, he gave gifts, money, and food to some of the poor around him.

Sisi spent her early days in the neighbourhood of Possenhofen, which her father owned. She was allowed plenty of time to play in the parks and playgrounds. Her childhood was happy, and she enjoyed horse riding and loved ordinary people. Her mother, however, seemed more focused on her older sister, Helene, and Sisi was often put on the back burner.

She had a much closer relationship with her father and brothers as she shared her father's love of nature and the mountains. At age five, Sisi had a governess whom she managed to wrap around her finger, often managing to avoid her studies. She learned to swim and ride her little pony along with her father's bigger horses. One day she was thrown from one of his large, untrained horses, much to the horror of her governess. But Sisi quickly brushed it aside and hopped back on. She often enjoyed riding through the Alps with her father, where they would rest in Chalets, enjoying food and music together.

When it was arranged that the emperor of Austria, Franz Joseph, was to meet Sisi's sister Helene for a marriage contract, things took a different turn. As we learned earlier, Sophia wanted a niece from the House of Wittelsbach to marry her son, as the Houses of Wittelsbach and Habsburg were two of the oldest ruling houses in Europe. Both were staunch Catholics, and previous centuries of inbreeding had already brought the two families together.

When the families agreed to meet on 16 August in Ischl, it was Sisi, not her sister, that Franz Joseph noticed. She entered the room, holding a bunch of wild roses, wearing a beautiful white dress, with her long brown hair falling over her youthful figure.

'I am Elisabeth!' the fifteen-year-old girl boldly introduced herself and Franz Joseph was immediately taken by her beautiful blue eyes.

He had never been overly worried about marriage, but everything changed when he laid eyes on Sisi. He announced that he would marry no other. Sisi certainly wasn't his mother's first choice, but she figured it might be easier to manipulate her over her older sister.

Though Sisi felt she was a bit young for marriage, she happily agreed to marry her cousin. The people of Vienna were delighted and soon poems were being written about her loveliness.

On 20 April 1854, Elisabeth of Bavaria began her journey to Vienna, and she was overwhelmed by how much her own people celebrated along with her. The following day, her barge travelled down the Danube, where her future husband greeted her once she entered the city. She was again overcome with joy, not only at the delight of her people, but those of the city of Vienna as well. She was received with a warm welcome.

When Elisabeth made her way to Vienna to get married, her coach was drawn by eight white horses, a coachman and a footman dressed in elaborate white wigs. She wore a pale pink gown embroidered in silver. Diamonds were strewn throughout her hair, along with white and pink roses. Close to 7,000 people gathered for the royal wedding that took place on 24 April 1854. When the Archbishop announced their marriage, a thundering of gunfire was heard around them. On the wedding day, Franz Joseph was so overcome with emotion that he pardoned almost every case of high treason in the courts as well as most general offences against the public. It is said that on the wedding day, Elisabeth of Bavaria was the loveliest empress the Habsburgs had ever seen. They were entranced by her deep blue eyes, fair complexion, and long chestnut-coloured hair.

While the middle-class Austrians were delighted with Sisi, some aristocrats were not. Some felt she was too young and not distinguished enough to be their empress. Sisi found rules at the Austrian Court to be petty and ridiculous. She refused the hot dishes laid before her at many of the daily luncheons, instead asking for a glass of Munich beer with bread and sausage. This appalled many around her. She also breached etiquette by removing her gloves at a court reception and said it was ridiculous that anyone should be offended by such a thing. But because Franz Joseph was so very much in love with his new wife, he allowed her to relax some of the rigid and more ancient customs at court.

Sisi found herself having to contend with her power-hungry mother-in-law, who made it clear that she was in charge at Court. She had a lot of influence over her son, and it was very difficult for the two strong-minded women to get along. Sisi came to court with the impression that she would be the number one woman in her husband's life, but she was often pushed away by Sophia. The actions of her mother-in-law put an automatic strain on the couple, often leaving Sisi overcome with melancholy. These feelings of depression were soon followed by coughing fits, anxiety, and a sense of fear.

When the couple's first daughter was born in March 1855, ten months after the wedding day, her mother-in-law named the baby Sophia, after herself, without consulting either parent. She also refused to let Elisabeth nurse her baby, likely leading to her becoming pregnant again soon after. A second daughter, Archduchess Gisela of Austria, born in 1856, also immediately taken from the room by Sophia, referring to Sisi as a 'silly, young mother'.[1] Franz was likely torn on what to do but refused to go against anything his mother did. Sophie also told her daughter-in-law that her failure to produce a male heir made her worthless.

In 1857, the family of four travelled to Hungary, and Sisi fell in love with the country and its people. However, both her children fell ill with diarrhoea, and little Gisela (1856–1932) recovered, but Sophia (1855–1887) lost her life at only two years old. On the couple's return to Vienna, Sophia said that her granddaughter's death was proof that Sisi was an unfit mother, and this only caused Sisi's depression to deepen.

The empress was still loved by the townsfolk with great measure and spent much of her early years of marriage mingling with them as she walked through the city streets, shopped in boutiques, and met with the large crowds that surrounded her. She was just as smitten with them as they were with her. She dazzled those from other countries as well, and on a trip to Milan, Franz Joseph told her: 'Your charm has done more to win over these people than all my soldiers with their bayonets and cannons could possibly affect.'[2]

Finally, on the evening of 21 August 1858, Sisi gave birth to the long-awaited heir. Everyone was delighted and poured into the churches to pray for mother and child. They named the child Rudolph (1858–1889). Of his son Franz Joseph said:

> Heaven has sent me a son who will one day see a new larger, and more beautiful city. But whatever changes there may be in the capital, the prince will always find the old loyal hearts, who, if it should ever prove necessary, will devote themselves to his cause under all circumstances.[3]

It seemed that the queen mother was finally satisfied with Sisi, but this baby was also taken to a nursery at the far end of the castle where he was out of his mother's reach. Sisi begged to be able to have her son with her, but this only angered her mother-in-law. As far as Sophia was concerned, Sisi had done her job and was of little to no importance anymore.

Sisi was overwhelmed with anxiety about how destructive her mother-in-law's power over her husband was in every aspect, even politics. When war broke out between France and Sardinia in 1959, and Sisi devoted herself to visiting the sick and wounded soldiers of the Italian army, we have to wonder if it was her way of coping with Sophia. She made her way to every soldier she could in the hospitals, offering kind words and gifts.

The treatment from her mother-in-law began to drain her, and her relationship with her husband began to sour as a result. She became distant, withdrawn and filled with scorn, which caused him to neglect her even more. Courtiers began to feel disdain for her again, and she began to feel self-conscious. Her health began to suffer, and she soon became ill. Her doctors concluded that she was suffering from a lung infection, and she was encouraged to visit the island of Madeira, which was said to be the best place for those with consumption. She put this off until early 1861, but her long illness had ravaged her, and she sank deeper into a depression. Some feared she might not even survive the journey.

But she did survive and found the island to be warm with tropical fruits, sunshine and clear skies, a huge relief from the fog and cold of Vienna. Her rooms were lovely, with a large veranda, beautiful furniture, and a mountain view. Her terrace also overlooked the sea. There were flowers in the gardens, and she enjoyed the outdoors very much. Perhaps it reminded her of her childhood love for the outdoors and the time she had spent with her father. Sisi found that she loved being away from court even though she was sick. She reflected on her Bavarian people and her childhood home. She wrote to her family often, enjoyed nature, and read for countless hours a day.

After four months her coughing fits became less frequent and less severe, and so she returned to Vienna. Her vessel home hit a bad storm and was thrashed around violently, but Sisi insisted she remain on deck and seemed almost to enjoy the waves crashing over her.

She arrived in Trieste, where she was met by her husband, but just a few weeks after arriving home, she began to weaken and to cough again. She also developed horrible migraines. Her childhood doctor was consulted and said that Sisi had a serious internal complaint, though little details were given. This time she was sent to the island of Corfu to recover. She enjoyed the climate there even more than Madeira and again began to feel better. She fell in love with the island and spent much time in its small chapel. After a few months, doctors said she was nearly recovered, and in October she went to Venice to finish recuperating. Again, the people of Italy loved her.

When she returned to Vienna in 1862, the public once again welcomed her back. She chose to stay away from court for a time, but this upset her husband, who claimed he missed her company and that he was also concerned about their son's health. Sisi, too, softened towards her husband and finally returned to court to be with him. Although she was still struggling with depression, she continued to spend her time visiting wounded soldiers in hospitals, where she became known as the 'angel of the wounded.'

One day while sitting with a soldier with a serious head wound, he said: 'I have had the happiness to see my Empress by my deathbed, and there is nothing else to wish for in this world. Now I am content to die.'[4]

Sisi also strongly desired to restore peace between Austria and Hungary. She participated in the Austrian Hungarian Compromise of 1867, where a dual monarchy was established between the two countries. She and her husband were crowned king and queen of Hungary and given a new residence outside Budapest. It was here she gave birth to her daughter, Marie Valarie (1868–1924) on 22 April 1868

The people of Hungary were delighted. Sisi immediately bonded with her new baby as she refused to let her be taken by her mother-in-law. At the time, Rudolph was around 10 years old and still under the tutelage of his grandmother, which had made him into a vain little boy, much to Sisi's dismay. A few years later in 1872 however, the queen mother died.

Little Marie Valerie had inherited her mother's love of flowers, and they enjoyed visiting the castle gardens together. Sisi wanted her daughter to share her own love of horse riding, but Marie Valerie preferred literature, art, and poetry.

Horse riding had become almost like a form of therapy for Sisi throughout her life. She loved the long rides and spent hours grooming her horses and always had a sugar cube in her pocket for a tasty treat for them. Her long rides through the Hungarian plains helped Sisi combat the gloomy moods which plagued her more and more over the years, and she wondered if she was creeping towards the edge of madness. The frequency of her nervous episodes increased, and she would often ride for miles during the early dawn or dusk to escape from other people and everything that worried her.

Sisi also developed a fondness for dressing in plain clothes and getting to know the Hungarian people. It truly exhausted her to participate in public affairs as she didn't care for the noise or the excitement. Her frequent illnesses didn't help either. When she did have to obey her imperial duties and appear for public affairs, it made her miserable. She once said: 'My long isolation has taught me that the burden of existence becomes heaviest in the presence of our fellow beings.'[5]

The Viennese courtiers still had no great favour with Sisi, and when she was back at court, she befriended a small African boy who happily did her bidding. She was very kind to young Mahmoud and even nursed him back to health when he fell ill from consumption. Her daughter, Marie Valerie, became a childhood companion of the boy. The aristocrats were appalled at this, and when Sisi heard how offended they were, she purposely had her daughter and Mahmoud photographed together and exhibited the image. This caused even more evil tongues to wag, and people began to wonder if she had gone mad.

Despite the unkind words of those around her, Sisi's love of helping others remained consistent. She continued to visit patients who were in with typhus and cholera without a second thought as to whether she could get infected herself.

Young Rudolph had grown up as a student at the University of Vienna, where he studied the arts. He became close with his mother, and the two became good friends. When it came time for him to marry, Franz Joseph looked for a political match, but Sisi wanted him to be happy. Franz Joseph felt that the Belgian Princess Stephanie (1864–1945) would be a good match, and the two were married on 10 September 1881. Sisi wasn't overly fond of Stephanie as she disliked her father, the Belgian King Leopold II (1835–1909), and the relationship between Sisi and Rudolph became strained after he married.

Throughout her adult life, the empress suffered far more than her doctors realised. Towards the end of 1870, Sisi had common complaints of neurasthenia, which today would be known as fatigue, headache, and irritability. This was a hereditary issue within the House of Wittelsbach that showed up repeatedly in its members. Those affected showed a general preference for solitude, were not terribly interested in mixing with large crowds and found themselves almost continuously restless. All these traits were clearly inherited by Sisi.

With the development of sudden rheumatism in her knees, she had been forced to give up her love for riding, which devastated her. She also had debilitating sciatica, causing her to cry out when the pain got unbearable.

But despite her pain, Sisi bore her discomfort almost heroically and took up walking and hiking as an alternative to her beloved riding. She still longed to get outdoors and appeared to have good stamina when it came to her walks and hikes through the mountains. Perhaps it was the constant excitement of her nerves that kept her moving. Or perhaps it was because she suffered so terribly from insomnia that she was desperate to exhaust herself physically in the hope that she might sleep.

Sisi also grew to have a very simple diet and a small appetite. She hardly ate at social events, even large banquets with an array of food. Her meals often consisted of nothing more than a piece of bread, some broth, and a piece of fruit. She usually ate a piece of bread, a biscuit, and a glass of milk at dinner.

She sometimes went weeks, even months, drinking only milk and oranges as she was terrified of gaining weight. She admired her tiny physique and felt that being very thin was the epitome of health. At 5ft 8in, Sisi never weighed more than 8 stone, except during pregnancy. Her exercise routines included using gymnasium mats and balance beams, and she kept her waist around 16 inches for most of her life. She weighed herself almost daily, and if she had gained even a pound, she reverted to her orange and milk diet until she was again comfortable with her desired weight. She seldom drank alcohol, even when a glass of wine was prescribed as a means of relaxation.

She may not have eaten much herself, but when it came to friends and family visiting court, she went out of her way to ensure they were served an array of beautiful and well-prepared dishes – thought she never enjoyed them herself. Sisi had very little faith in doctors of the time and preferred her own methods to treat herself, which greatly irritated her doctors.

Aside from her husband and family, Sisi kept her distance from most at court, and if servants or courtiers didn't respect her wishes for solitude, she would get furious. In one case, she boxed the ears of a gentleman servant, witnessed by several people. Because of her history of kindness towards others, this must have been a sure sign of her increasing depression and misery.

After Sisi's death, the following was written about her by another of her ladies:

'We who loved her so well and knew her so intimately, just because we were so devoted to her, cannot speak of her. Our voices are choked with tears. She was one of those exceptional characters who are independent of the world because they are within themselves a life richer and better than that of ours. Every thought and instinct were on a higher level. She was inanimately a queen. And yet she was always modest, simple, thoroughly human, and full of touching consideration towards all in attendance upon her. Indeed, her thoughtfulness often distressed them, for she refrained from ringing in the night, though racked with pain because she would not deprive others of their rest. A consideration frequently unknown to the empress included some of her ladies watching through the night outside the door of her room.

We went to her with our deepest thoughts as well as our most worldly concerns, always confident of her every ready sympathy, her tender council or prompt assistance in case of need.'

From as early as anyone could remember, Sisi had been blessed with divine beauty and intellect, which was rare for someone who carried several defective genes due to family inbreeding. No one at court seemed to have more grace than Sisi. Even though she preferred modest clothing, she was always a sight to behold. When she reached the age of 50, it is said she didn't look older than 20. Sisi's hair had always been of her best attributes, falling to her knees in long chestnut waves. But while others felt she wore her hair like an angel's halo, she was often bothered by it, especially when she got older, and was most bothered by any signs of grey hair. She once stated that her hair was like a 'heavy, foreign object upon her head'. Once while being tended to, she told her lady: 'I am nothing but a slave to my hair and perhaps I shall cut every bit of it off.'

But she would never do such a thing. A tent had been erected on the terrace of her palace where she could have her hair dressed in full view of the open sea.

Sometimes, in the dead of night, after everyone at court had retired for the evening, Sisi would wander the palace grounds, dressed in black with a black veil covering her face. When she went for hikes in the mountains, she chose the steepest and most dangerous paths and never took any ladies with her. The stillness of the mountains, the clean air, and the beauty of nature seemed to bring some peace to her restless spirit. She once claimed:

'I wish for nothing from mankind except be left in peace.'

And yet, despite this, Sisi still loved nothing more than spending time with the commoners, and it seemed they understood her kind heart and gentle nature. When she was seen in public, people would cross themselves, men would admire her, and children would stand in awe to look at her.

On 31 January 1889, tragedy struck. Sisi's son, Rudolph, the Crown Prince, was found dead in his bed at his imperial hunting lodge in Mayerling, Austria, where he spent a few days with his lover, the Baroness Mary Vetsera (1871–1889). They were both found dead as either a murder-suicide or a suicide pact. The consensus was that it was suicide, but some historians believe it was murder. However, like his mother, Rudolph was loved by the people, so it was difficult to fathom that someone would want him dead.

Terror swept over the capital of Austria when Rudolph's death was announced. The empress was the first one to hear the news. Rudolph's gentleman-in-waiting was very distraught about delivering the news to Sisi, knowing how fragile she already was. When the empress was told, she went silent for several minutes before asking, 'Where is my son?'

She then began talking about how to tell Franz Joseph, as he was not yet aware of the news and was determined to be the one to deliver the news to him. She stood by her husband faithfully through the entire ordeal and was nothing but tender and kind. She tried desperately not to show her grief in front of her husband so she could instead focus on his.

Of his wife's support, Franz Joseph said: 'I cannot describe in adequate words my deep gratitude to my dearly loved consort who has proved herself a strong support during these sorrowful days, and I devoutly thank God for giving me such a helpmate. Repeat my words, for the wider you spread them abroad, the more heartily thankful I shall feel.'[6]

The hope of an heir to the throne had been ripped from the emperor and empress in the blink of an eye, and their sorrow was shared from Budapest to Vienna as the royal couple was met with nothing but condolences.

Elizabeth said of her son's passing: 'There is a moment in the life of each one where the spirit dies and by no means follows that this need be at the time of the physical death.'[7]

The death of Rudolph would change Empress Elisabeth forever. She was never heard laughing again, and rarely smiled. Her shock and bravery for her husband eventually wore off, and she fell into total despair. She said she had 'no longer either the strength to live and the wish to die'.[8]

Her sobs of misery were heard by all who attended her, and her aversion to the world became even more pronounced as her absence from court became more frequent. She refused to see her daughter-in-law or grandchildren, for she could not look at her granddaughter, who looked so much like Rudolph.

Along with her deepening melancholy, her doctors had also discovered that she had been suffering from heart disease (although one could always hypothesise that she was suffering from a broken heart). She became more of a stranger to people and rarely visited Vienna anymore. Her social circle became smaller and smaller. She shut people out and gave orders that no one should be able to view her in public.

Elisabeth stopped visiting her favourite castle in Lainz, her passion for travel began to diminish, and she concluded that she felt trapped as if she were a caged animal. Franz Joseph often came to see his wife but found it hard to pull her from the trenches of melancholy she had fallen into. She continued to grieve terribly and was a shadow of who she had been.

In 1890, Sisi's older sister Helene died; that same year, Marie Valerie married Francis Salvator, the Duke of Tuscany (1866–1939). Despite her misery, the empress put a smile on her face for her daughter's wedding, but it was short-lived. Inside, she felt even more saddened that her daughter would be leaving her to start her own life.

In late January of 1892, her mother, who had always been a nurturing friend to her, also died, pulling Sisi deeper into depression. She withdrew to her castle in Corfu, where she erected a monument to her beloved son, and seemed only to exist in her mind, reliving her memories of him. In the mountains of Aja Kyriahi, a tiny church was erected that she visited every morning before sunrise with the explicit orders that no one else be there at that time. She wandered alone through some of the more dangerous paths through the mountains, wallowing in her misery. On the interior walls of the church, this inscription was found:

> I can breathe with greater freedom on these lonely heights where others would feel themselves forsaken. I am perfectly satisfied on Aja Kyriahi and could even renounce my passion for travelling if I could remain on its heights forever.[9]

The empress was only seen for a few hours a day by her ladies as she seemed to be living in a dream world, reading Shakespeare, and recreating the playwright's characters in her head as she imagined they were coming alive before her.

On a rare occasion, she did appear at court to visit with the Tsar and Tsarina of Russia, Nicholas, and Alexandra. Sisi was received at the gala reception on the arm of the Tsar, still looking like she was in mourning.

In 1896, Hungary celebrated the royal couple's millenary. The empress was miserable and had no desire to attend, but also did not want to let her people down. She sat on her throne next to her husband, dressed in black with a veil over her hair. Her face was pale white and almost unrecognisable. When the President of the Chamber spoke, Elisabeth was indifferent and expressionless. When her name was mentioned, she didn't seem to register, though her eyes did tear up in response to the applause she received from the Hungarian people. Little did they know, this would be the last time she would appear in the country.

Towards the latter years of her life, Sisi made it clear that she had no fear of dying: 'I am ready to die. My only wish is that I may be spared acute and lingering suffering.'[10]

It seemed that Elisabeth fantasised about odd manners of death, such as when she walked by the sea with one of her ladies, she was quoted saying, 'The sea is longing to have me, and I know that I belong to it. What does it matter if I am drowned?'[11]

She developed bizarre beauty rituals, washing her hair in cognac and egg yolk, showering in frigid water in the morning, and taking olive oil baths in the evening. She slept with a leather facemask filled with crushed strawberries and raw veal. She had decided that her image of public beauty must never change, and she refused any more portraits or photographs.

Her husband felt that she was creeping closer and closer to insanity, as her expression was always restless. A constant frown had developed and, in turn, harsh frown lines around her mouth. She suffered from almost constant nerve pain throughout her whole body. Franz noticed that she was deathly thin, and her hands shook so much that she didn't want to be around him or her children. It was only in the summer of 1898 when she went to Ischl to celebrate her husband's birthday, that she did not wear mourning clothes while attending a church service.

Her doctors instructed her to go to Manheim in Hesse to rest, and before she left, the papers in Austria and Hungary stated:

> Her Majesty, the Empress and Queen has been suffering for some long time past from anaemia which became worse in consequence of severe neuritis in the course of last winter, following on insomnia of many weeks standing in addition to which there is an enlargement of the heart. Under conditions of absolute rest, her illness need not give rise to serious apprehensions, but the doctors earnestly advise Her Majesty to submit to treatment of the baths in order to strengthen the muscles of her heart.[12]

One evening in Manheim, she was eating a peach when a raven swooped down and grabbed it. Her lady was very nervous because the Habsburgs had always viewed the raven as a bad omen. But Sisi was not bothered, saying: 'Dear Friend, I fear nothing. What is to be will be, and I am a fatalist.'[13]

In September 1889, Sisi travelled to Switzerland and stayed in a Geneva hotel where the local police were instructed to watch over her. Of course, as usual, Sisi stated she just wanted to be left alone. On the way to board a steamship, she passed a man sitting on a bench on the Quai Montblanc. The man was Luigi Luccheni (1873–1910), an Italian activist who was known to authorities.

Luccheni lunged at Sisi, and one of her ladies caught her as she collapsed, asking if she was ill. Sisi replied that she did not know, before becoming very pale. She continued to make her way onto the ship before falling again and fainting. Her lady and some of the ship's staff loosened her coat to give her some air as it was a hot day. It was then that they discovered the blood seeping through her blouse. Luccheni had stabbed Sisi in the chest with what was later discovered to be a four-inch filing needle.

'What has happened?' the empress asked. Those would be her last words.

The steamship returned to shore, and she was taken to the hospital, where she died after taking two deep breaths.

Only a few days earlier, Sisi had remarked to one of her ladies that, 'I should like to have a quick, painless death, not to die in my bed.'[14]

The empress got her to wish as her doctors concluded that her death was quick and painless.

Of her death, Franz Joseph said, 'She has done good to many but no harm to a single human being. Nobody can conceive the magnitude of the loss I have sustained. Not one blow has spared me in this world. Without her, I should never have been able to carry out the work which God has laid upon my shoulders.'

Sisi was misunderstood to the last hour of her life and was judged for the innate tendencies of the Wittelsbach empire. However, throughout her life, Sisi shared a common bond with her cousin, King Ludwig II, who also struggled tremendously with mental illness.

The disabling trait of mental illness certainly didn't discriminate when it came to members of the royal Wittelsbachs – for the unfortunate gene also caught Sisi's cousin, King Ludwig II of Bavaria, in its web. Ludwig, like his cousin, was the result of the intermarriage that had long been entangling the royal family.

Ludwig's father, Maximillian II of Bavaria (1811–1864), married his cousin, Marie of Prussia (1825–1889), in October 1842. While she was a Protestant, Maximillian was a staunch Catholic. Marie was very beautiful with raven hair and huge blue eyes, and along with her good looks, went her charm. Maximillian, who was generally well-liked as a monarch, also may have suffered from mental illness during his life.

On 25 August 1845, physicians and close family surrounded Marie in her apartments as she went into labour with her first child. Despite concerns about her small pelvis, she delivered a son on Saint Ludwig's Day. The child was born at 12.30 pm at Nymphenburg Palace in Munich, sporting the same black hair and deep blue eyes as his mother. Since 1715, Nymphenburg Palace has served as the summer residence of electors and kings of the House of Wittelsbach.

Maximillian's father, Ludwig I, was so delighted with the birth of his grandson that he was soon embracing everyone around him. Because the child was born on Saint Ludwig's day, his grandfather thought the name Ludwig was only fitting. A 101-gun salute announced the birth of Ludwig the following day, shortly followed by his baptism.

While Ludwig may have been predisposed to mental illness, we can not overlook the tragedies that bestowed his early life, which must have in some way contributed to his eventual downfall. When he was only 8 months old, his wet nurse died of typhoid, and he was suddenly weaned from the breast, causing him to become ill. He was probably faced with his first bout of real shock.

As a young child, Ludwig was shy and introverted and preferred playing on his own instead of with others. He was given a toy replica of the Arch of Victory, a three-arched memorial crowned with a statue of Bavaria with a lion quadriga. He was enthralled with it, and it's possible that the gift was what sparked Ludwig's love of building.

From the age of 8, the young prince was given regular lessons from tutors, including writing and religious instruction. His handwriting was exceptionally meticulous and ornate. It would be for most of his life until his mental illness became so profound that his penmanship was reduced to something almost unreadable. Michael Klass, Ludwig's German mentor, wanted him to be raised healthy and with strong Christian values.

One of the most impressionable people in his early life was his governess, Fraulein Meilhause, whom he cared for very deeply. Frau Meilhause was known for her gentleness and way of conveniently overlooking any of Ludwig's faults. However, in 1854, Ludwig had to part with his governess in favour of a new governor, Count Theodor Basselet de La Rosee (1801–1864). Parting with his beloved governess caused great sadness in Ludwig, and he soon began to feel the icy cold grip of anxiety. Already, he had lost his wet nurse, whom he undoubtedly bonded with as an infant. And now the woman who was more of a mother figure to him was also taken. Because Frau Meilhaus had been so devoted to the prince, he must have felt like he had lost his mother.

Summer and fall for Ludwig and his younger brother, Otto, born three years after Ludwig, were spent in Hohenschwangau Castle and Berchtesgaden Castle. Hohenschwangau was built by Ludwig's father, and Berchtesgaden Castle was used primarily as a hunting lodge for the royal family. The brothers were kept under the watchful eye of their new governor, who was quite conventional and only wanted the boys to play with other noble children. He ordered everyone to bow to the Crown Prince, but Bavarian rule stated that this was not necessary until he had reached the age of 18. Instead, de La Rossee singled the prince out, causing Ludwig to lose favour with him as he was too overbearing.

In 1855, both boys were given a military instructor, Baron Emil Von Wulffen (1828–1876) and a new, more strenuous plan was put in place. Von Wulffen said Ludwig should 'learn to think' and become more psychically fit. This new plan was based on that of his cousin, Franz Joseph, who, at the time, was the future emperor of Austria and would become Empress Elisabeth's husband, as we learned earlier. With these new plans in place, Ludwig was instructed to study from 5.30 every morning until 8.30 in the evening. This rigorous new schedule caused Ludwig to feel a considerable amount of stress, and he was rarely able to spend much time outside playing with his brother, Otto (1848–1911). The two liked to play dress-up and recreate scenes from history.

During the fall of 1857, a strange incident occurred, which might possibly give the first clue that Ludwig was mentally unstable. The brothers were playing in the park at Berchtesgaden when Ludwig suddenly held his brother down, binding his hands and feet and then gagging him. He put a handkerchief around his neck and twisted it tight with a stick, creating a tourniquet. When the boys were discovered, Ludwig said: 'He is my vassal. It is none of your business.'[15]

Ludwig then had to endure a proper beating from his enraged father. Was Ludwig re-enacting a scene from history, or perhaps one from his beloved plays?

Germans were turned off by French literature after the revolution, and many turned to their own country's legends of dark gods, brace knights, maidens, dragons and being who were half-man and half-beast. Ludwig soon became obsessed with these playwrights, especially the work of Richard Wagner (1813–1883). Wagner was a German composer and theatre director known especially for his eccentric operas. His fantasy-based works fascinated Ludwig, especially in his malleable adolescent years, and unlike most Germans, Ludwig had a liking for French culture. His grandfather, Ludwig I, was a godson of Marie Antionette, the ill-fated queen of France. While he, of course, never met her, Ludwig developed a deep passion for her, calling her 'la sainte reine' or 'the holy queen'.

Aside from his fantasies about Marie Antionette, Prince Ludwig was quite the daydreamer, yet those around him, especially his tutors, seemed oblivious. Often gifted with portraits of saints and busts of

Goethe and Schiller, both German composers, Ludwig was delighted. Ludwig was also fascinated by the Oberammergau, a seventeenth-century play depicting the passion of Christ.

Another of Ludwig's enthusiasms in life lay with his cousin, Sisi. They had adored each other since childhood, and though she was eight years older than him, they would have a profound lifelong connection to one another. It was a connection that surpassed friendship and even love, as both were enthralled by the magnificent things in life and profoundly romantic at heart. It's possible that Ludwig's feelings went a bit further for his cousin, for in his mind, she was the incarnation of the beloved Marie Antionette. Like Sisi, Ludwig also had a true love of the Bavarian people and loved to spend time with the peasants and farmers.

Ludwig also became very close to his cousin Anna, Princess of Hesse and the Rhine (1843–1865), the daughter of his aunt, Elizabeth of Prussia (1815–1885). The Bavarian Royal House was closely allied with the Grand Ducal House of Hesse-Darmstadt by both blood and marriage.

But it was Ludwig's love for Wagner that would surpass all. Wagner's play *Lohengrin*, first performed in 1850, depicted a mysterious knight who comes by swan boat to help a distressed noble lady. When Ludwig first saw the play, it was the most spiritual and emotional thing that had ever happened to him.

As a child, Ludwig constantly felt as if he were being watched, which he undoubtedly was, leading to him being highly strung and nervous. With his excessive imagination, Ludwig often felt he was treated like a cornered animal with no way out. But upon seeing the fearless knight of the swan in Wagner's play, it became like the personification of his inner struggles against humiliation. He also developed an obsession with Wagner's four-part opera depicting German Folklore, *Nibelungen*, which premiered in 1869. He was enchanted with Wagner's *Work of the Art of the Culture*.

As Ludwig's intense education continued, La Rossee felt it was time to make some changes. He demanded that Ludwig discontinue his piano lessons because he would never be any good at it. He also thought the prince should stop learning Greek and should learn how to properly use weapons.

While Ludwig was soon becoming an incredibly handsome Crowned Prince, he was also frequently ill. In early August of 1862, he wrote to his cousin Anna:

> Because of my sore throat, I am not allowed to make long excursions. I also had to give up horseback riding. A doctor from Berlin, Dr Traute, examined me. At the beginning, it was rather frightening. I was conducted into a dark room, and there he looked into my throat with a mirror. But he only found a slight enlargement of the larynx. But he is a Jew, and his looks are not very taking.[16]

While this letter speaks of a mild illness, it also gives our first clue that Ludwig would base much of what he thought he knew on how people looked.

On his 17th birthday, he was made a knight of the ancient Wittelsbach Family Order of Saint Hubertus, and when he turned 18 in August of 1863, he was given two orderly officers and several domestic male servants. He also had to go to Munich to see his cousin, the king of Prussia. One of the king's gentlemen, Prince Kraft Hohenlohe Ingelfingen (1827–1892), had a very favourable impression of Ludwig: 'Everyone admired his brilliance, physical skill, courage and great understanding of art and science.'[17]

Another of the Prussian king's men, Minister Bismarck (1815–1898), said:

> It seemed to me that his thoughts were away from the table, and only now and again did he remember his intention to talk to me. But even so, I recognised a talent, a vivacity and good sense. In some conversations, he looked up at the ceiling and continued to empty his champagne glass.

His surroundings seemed to bore him, and the champagne seemed to aid in the play of his independent fantasy.[18]

After several days in Munich, Ludwig composed a letter to his prior governess, with whom he had still maintained a relationship. Addressing her now as Frau Von Leonrod, he told her of a man who had won his heart, the third son of Maximilian Karl, 6th Prince of Thurn and Taxis, Paul of Taxis (1843–1879). Maximillian married Helene of Bavaria, Sisi's sister and Ludwig's cousin.

The Thurn and Taxis family owned a palace in Regensburg, a city in eastern Bavaria, and several other castles and properties. The family was hereditary Postmaster General to the empire and had great wealth. Sources say that Paul was charming, good looking and easily fell under Ludwig's spell of seduction. Paul was Ludwig's first real friend as they played together as children with Sisi and her siblings.

Ludwig wrote several letters to his cousin, Anne, suggesting a strong intimacy between him and Paul. Both men were young, romantically minded and enjoyed nature. During the fall of 1863, he spent nearly all of his time with Paul, and Paul's letter to Ludwig made their relationship clear: 'During the day and especially in the evenings, I miss very much your visits and how often I would like to be near you in order to calm you and prevent you from getting too intense and passionate and in a state of excitement about our affair.'[19]

But court and government officials were less than happy about the budding romance between the two men. Ludwig was of an age where he had royal duties, and his days needed to be planned to the minute. A letter to Ludwig from Paul reflects this:

> I often think of what you are doing and wonder whether you think of me. Please do write to me as I am always much happier when I know that you are happy, healthy, and living on good terms with yourself and your

surroundings. I always wear your chain and consider it a symbol of the faith with which our friendship is bound together.[20]

Not many other letters between the two men have been found as it is believed that all of them, along with any evidence of Pauls' relationship with the prince, was destroyed by Paul's family.

At 11.45 on the morning of 10 March 1864, Ludwig's father, King Maximillian II, died in his sleep of a short and unexpected illness. Much like his son, he was also physically delicate, as were so many in the Wittelsbach dynasty. He was plagued with headaches and nervousness and showed signs of mental illness towards the end of his life. He was buried on 14 March, and Bavaria had a new king.

Ludwig II, the new Bavarian king, was 18 years old, 6ft 3in tall, and very handsome. He had a beautiful face, ivory skin, jet black hair, and sharp blue pensive eyes. An Austrian writer said of the new king:

He was the most beautiful youth I have ever seen. His tall, slim figure was perfectly symmetrical. His rich, slightly curling hair and the few traces of a moustache gave his head a similarity to those great antique works of art through which we have our first idea of Hellenic manly strength. Even if he had been a beggar, I would have noticed him. Nobody, old or you, rich or poor, could be left untouched by his charm, which radiated from his personality. His voice was agreeable. The questions which he asked were clear and definitive. The subject of his conversations was well-chosen and spiritual. He expressed himself with ease and naturally. The enthusiasm with which he inspired me never diminished but, only the contrary, increased with the years.[21]

As king, Ludwig declared that he would 'do everything in my power to make my people happy. Their welfare, their peace, are the conditions of my own happiness.'[22]

However, one of the first things Ludwig did as king was summon Wagner, aged 50, to Munich. He wrote a letter to him, saying that ever since he saw the production of *Lohengrin*, he was enchanted with his music. He said he had dreamt of him, read his books with pleasure, and his greatest wish was to meet him. He also sent along a photo and a gold ring set with a ruby.

Wagner, who had been in considerable debt for a long time, saw the king's letter as a true miracle. He went to see him the next day, his train arriving in Munich at 10.30 pm. He was received by His Majesty the following afternoon, and the two seemed to appreciate one another. While Wagner may have been more in love with the idea of having his debt paid off, Ludwig fell in love with Wagner at first sight, even going so far as to hug him when they met. While Wagner was not tall and looked a bit hunchbacked, Ludwig saw only beauty.

It's worth taking a moment to delve deeper into what 'in love' meant for the king. It was clear by now that Ludwig preferred the company of men over women, at least in terms of attraction. While he favoured Sisi and was in awe of Marie Antoinette, we can not say he was romantically in love with them. It's possible to say this for Paul of Taxis, as it was certainly suggestive in their letters. As for Wagner, was Ludwig really in love with him, or was he in love with who he was; the poet, the composer, the magician that seemed able to reach deep into Ludwig's troubled mind with his music? Wagner was most certainly bisexual as he had mistresses and took an interest in women. He had even been married but left the relationship when his finances fell into dire straits. But what would become of his new relationship with the king of Bavaria?

Wagner stayed in Munich for several days as the two became better acquainted. The king was romantic, sincere, and truthful, while Wagner was a realist. He could also be greedy and would gladly accept any financial help Ludwig offered him.

On 26 May 1864, Wagner penned a note to a friend of his, telling him of his experience: 'And then this charming care for me, this winning chastity of heart, of every feature. When he assures me of his happiness in possessing me. Thus, we sat for hours together, lost in each other's gaze.'[23]

Wagner never seemed to outwardly tell the king that he had an interest in women as well as men, and perhaps it is because he didn't want to jeopardise any monetary benefits he was getting out of the friendship. But like the king, he loved feminine things, such as perfumes and luxurious décor. He had also, on occasion, dressed as a woman. Like the king, everything that Wagner did had to be over the top. Wagner also had extreme political views, and the Bavarian people soon became concerned that their new king was falling under Wagner's influence. He had already spent a considerable number of years in exile in France and Switzerland due to his drastic beliefs. During the Dresden uprising of 1849, he had written several articles calling for a revolution. When the uprising failed, he fled the country to avoid an arrest warrant. The Bavarian people saw Wagner as a dangerous free spirit who could easily exploit their king as well as empty his bank account.

Yet, Ludwig didn't hesitate to give his new friend a private house with a beautiful garden in Munich along the royal avenue of Brienner Strasse. The house had coloured silk and lace upholstery, and the rooms were freshened with the smell of heavy perfumes, which reflected Wagner's love of such things. Both men were clearly egotistical and had little use for those who didn't minister to their vanity.

The king also allotted Wagner a healthy annual salary of 8,000 guilders which was paid in advance, along with helping him to pay off the mountain of debt he had accumulated over the years.

In July of 1864, Ludwig, met with Marie of Hesse and the Rhine (1824–1880), wife of Emperor Alexander II of Russia (1818–1881). The Empresses was hopeful that Ludwig would fall in love with her 10-year-old daughter, Grand Duchess Marie Alexandra (1853–1925).

But the Bavarian king had no interest in marriage – and just as well because his grandfather advised that he was much too young to be married and to enjoy his status as a bachelor. Most royal families were eager to arrange marriages for political reasons, so it must have been a bit of a relief that Ludwig's grandfather felt differently.

Clearly, the young king was more interested in decorating his rooms at Hohenschwangau Castle. His bedroom was decorated with scenes from *Jerusalem Delivered*, a sixteenth-century poem by Torquato Tasso. The poem told of a mythical and ornate version of the First Crusade. Tasso was also believed to have gone mad when he wrote the poem. The king also had orange trees painted on the blue ceilings, and a real fountain was constructed in part of his room. He had already planned for more orange trees and a moon to be painted on the walls. Ludwig also put in place the plans for a new national theatre, which Wagner had attempted to build earlier while still living in Dresden.

At the beginning of 1865, Ludwig I wrote to his grandson, counselling him not to let his new position overwhelm him and to try to relax in the evenings. Little did he know, the king wasn't working nearly that hard. Instead of worrying about the good of Bavaria, he was spending his time worrying about plays and poems. It was evident that Ludwig was having more and more bouts of escaping to a dream world: 'One of the greatest enjoyments of the mind is to be carried away by these wonderful works, and then elevated and strengthened one can face the realities of life again.'[24]

A letter from Austrian negotiator Count Blome written to Karl Ferdinand von Buol (1797–1865), the Austrian foreign minister, says this about the inattentive king:

> If I judge the young prince correctly, I should say that nature has endowed him with more imagination than brains and his boyhood heart was more neglected than anything...literary men and artistic are received in audience more than any other class of the population. His

Majesty's chief tastes lie in music and literature, more because of the words than the music itself.[25]

It was also in 1865 that Ludwig learned of Wagner's mistress, Cosima (1837–1930). It must have been a complete shock to him to realise that he was not the composer's one and only. Cosima was invited to Munich, and when she arrived, rumours began to fly that she was pregnant with Wagner's child. Upon hearing this, the king refused to go to a showing of Wagner's opera, *The Flying Dutchman,* or the showing of *Tannhauser*, another of his works. During the time of Cosima's visit, the king refused to see Wagner at all.

It's entirely possible that Ludwig was somehow perplexed by his friend. He was the one true love of Ludwig's life, yet there is no solid evidence suggesting that they had a serious physical relationship. We also aren't sure how well Wagner understood Ludwig's bizarre temperament. He fully understood that Ludwig preferred the company of men, as he knew of his prior relationship with Paul of Taxis. Yet, there is documentation of Wagner's writing of 'failing to understand how anyone could be homosexual'.[26]

Twenty-one years after Ludwig died, during a post-mortem exam,[27] doctors discovered that the first signs of mental illness were traceable to around 1865. Is it possible that discovering Cosima was the beginning of a breaking point for the king? Many people during his time thought he might be a simpleton because he had uncontrolled emotions, but Ludwig II was extremely bright from what we can understand.

As the king regressed further into his own world, the people began to refer to him as 'The Fairy King' due to his obsession with mythical creatures. He also began to spend more and more time away from Munich and court life. He made more and more trips into the mountains, where he built a small house where he could escape to. Like Sisi and most of the Wittelsbach family, the king could happily live in a palace or a peasant's inn, and it seemed to make no difference. He grew closer to his mother during his time away, as she also preferred isolation, flowers, and nature.

During the summer of 1865, Ludwig told his mother in a letter: 'More than anything, I like to be alone, occupy myself, and think of you and of Father, whom I imagine I see everywhere here. I am glad about this because every tree reminds me of him.'[28]

It seems this statement would stand out as a precursor to the hallucinations that would plague Ludwig later in his life.

In a letter written to the king that summer, Sisi seems to express her deep understanding of her cousin's condition, which was so much like her own:

> I am sorry beyond words that I have no chance of seeing
> you this summer. I understand only too well how much
> you need care and quietness after having been so ill last
> year. I need not tell you how vividly I am reminded of
> the many agreeable hours which I spent so happily with
> you last year.[29]

Ludwig spent the late part of that summer with Paul of Taxis and, on one particular day, dressed him up as Lohengrin, the legendary Knight of the Holy Grail. He was floated in a boat pulled by a fake swan for all to see, and this understandably gave way to a lot of gossip, giving the Bavarian people more reason to question their king's peculiar activities.

Swans filled Ludwig's life. Like the peacock that he loved, they were royal birds. At the age of five he was featured feeding swans with his mother, Queen Marie of Bavaria, and younger brother Prince Otto, in watercolour by E. Rietschel. At Hohenschwangau, the neo-Gothic castle of Ludwig's childhood, images of swans were on the walls, as was the legendary swan knight Lohengrin. There were porcelain swans at Neuschwanstein. Ludwig II would later be given a pair of swan cufflinks to Richard Wagner, his musical god. When he died, a Lohengrin costume was pathetically discovered among the clothing the king left behind.

After Cosima began writing to King Ludwig, asking for more money for herself and Wagner, Prime Minister Von der Pfordten threatened to resign if the king didn't part ways with the composer. Ludwig had no choice but to ask Wagner to leave Munich in late 1865.

In the summer of 1866, the Seven Weeks' War broke out as Prussia and Austria disputed over the governing of the Schleswig-Holstein area of Germany. But as the events leading up to the war developed, the king of Bavaria had more pressing matters to attend to.

The king and Paul of Taxis had fallen out of favour for a time, but in the spring of 1866, they began writing to one another again. These letters give an idea of how deep Ludwig's feelings went. They also tell us of the love triangle between himself, Paul, and Richard Wagner.

When Ludwig and Paul finally agreed to meet up in person, it was a very romantic encounter. The king had recently constructed a Winter Garden on the roof of the Munich Residenz, where the family usually resided in the colder months. The garden was only accessible from his private study, and he spent much time there entertaining guests. It was here that Paul and Ludwig met up, but not before this letter from Paul was sent to the king: 'Do let me assure you that you have found in me the most faithful and devoted friend who would rather lose his life and everything he possessed than you and your friendship.'[30]

After the two men met up, another of Paul's letters makes it clear just how much the friendship meant to him: 'I feel more closely bound together than ever before. Our relationship is now one of man-to-man. You are everything to me. May God give his blessing so that no power on earth may ever separate us.'[31]

These profound letters from Paul continued daily and were written almost as if they were two schoolgirls instead of grown men. Their relationship had reached a state of total euphoria.

And yet, despite this and the fact that Wagner had been asked to leave Munich, Ludwig still commanded him to come and perform *Lohengrin*, not caring what his critics said. The Bavarians were growing increasingly frustrated with their king because he didn't seem to care about politics at all. News of his correspondence with Wagner had leaked out, and the people once again disapproved, with many laying the blame directly on Wagner himself.

In a letter from Sisi to her mother, she said: 'I hear the king is away again. I wish he would care a little more about his duties, especially now when times are so bad.'[32]

But in May, as the threats of war were growing, the king was on a steamship with Paul, bound for Lake Lucerne in Switzerland, where they would stay at Wagner's villa. Plans were still in place for the Bavarian National Theatre and Opera House, and while at Wagner's home, the three men spent more time discussing and dreaming of the results. The king gave Paul the alias 'Friedrich', which would now be used in all further letters, probably to keep their relationship more concealed, whereas the king was not referred to as 'Most Beloved Angel'.

With Germany plunged into Civil War, in July of 1866, a telegraph was discovered that told of a discussion between the king, Paul and Wagner, stating that the king was considering abdication. But as we can assume, Wagner would have very little use for a throneless king. Paul was also very disturbed by his plans and wrote, telling him: 'You are destined to do great things, and only in your present position can you realise them and achieve greatness.'[33]

As part of trying to convince Ludwig of his importance, Paul urged him to visit the wounded soldiers and show them some compassion. Not surprisingly, Ludwig shied away from something so intimate and instead sent Paul on his behalf. And while his adversaries scrambled to form a peace treaty between Bavaria and Austria, the king was busy designing scenery and costumes for the upcoming Schiller play, *Wilhelm Tell*. He even went as far as parading around in the costumes and consuming great quantities of wine before heading off to state dinners.

And then, without much warning, Ludwig suddenly sent Paul away. Understandably, Paul was devastated and wrote Ludwig a tearful letter. Their relationship was that of a schoolboy fantasy, and Paul seemed to disappear from Ludwig's heart without warning.

In November of 1867, Ludwig became engaged to his first cousin, Duchess Sophie (1845–1921), the sister of Sisi, and the country was overjoyed. With Paul disgraced and Wagner still banned from Munich, Sophie suddenly filled an empty space in the king's life. They went to dances and balls together, but soon, like so many others, Sophie became like a romantic poetical phantom. Ludwig demanded she call him 'Heinrich', and she was now called 'Elsa', taking names from the Wagner's play Lohengrin. He was the eagle, and she was the dove.

It seemed as if Ludwig was intensely, even if briefly, infatuated with Sophie. After all, he'd certainly had those feelings for Sisi and Marie Antionette, at least in his mind. We could almost assume that Ludwig was forcing himself to believe he was in love, if only for the crown's sake. And yet, the shadow of Richard Wagner was ever-present. Every time that the king wrote to Sophie, Wagner was brought up. He even asked Sophie to write to Wagner herself; if possible, she should do so several times a day. Ludwig continuously invited her to have dinner with the two of them, referring to Wagner as 'The God of My Life'.

All of Ludwig's letters to Sophie were addressed to Elsa, and he would often complain about his aunt, Amalie of Greece, who was his father's sister-in-law: 'That plump bitch and interfering noodle ... a stout gossipy creature, the fat formless Greek majesty.'[34]

He also wrote to Sophie, asking to 'see the crown on her pretty head'.[35] And wrote of how a windstorm came through one evening while he was in his rooms. He pretended he was in Scotland with all his Scottish friends (which we aren't sure existed).

On 13 March 1867, Ludwig wrote to Sophie again, making Wagner the topic of conversation as well as his obsession with seeing the crown on her head:

> To nobody but you will I tell what I suffer. I am so truly happy about our engagement. But because the Precious Friend (Wagner) is here at the same time, I am utterly

unhappy and miserable. I entreat you. Do you make it possible for me to talk to him quietly? Nobody on earth could be possibly more precious to me. To think of the possibility of his death is unbearable. I would go mad.[36]

The king's emotions were so erratic and unstable that it must have been extremely confusing for his bride-to-be. The next morning, after writing the letter about his obsession with Wagner, he woke, overjoyed about seeing the ceremonial draft for their wedding. The wedding was to be on 25 August, the same day as Ludwig's 22nd birthday. But it was unexpectedly postponed until 12 October by Sophie's parents.

Understandably, Sisi was concerned about her cousin's sudden halt to the plans, and her parents intervened on her sister's behalf. Ludwig then wrote a curt note to Sophie: 'Your parents want to break off our engagement, and I accept the proposal.'[37]

He later wrote to her again, apologising for his rudeness, and told her she would always be in his heart. We can only imagine how she must have felt, to have been dropped so suddenly and unexpectedly by her fiancé. There were no warning signs, no suggestion that Ludwig was unhappy with the engagement. It was as if Ludwig's personality suddenly split into two, and Sophie was on the receiving end of the unkind one.

Sophie's brother, who was also Ludwig's cousin, wrote to him telling him that his behaviour was unforgivable. Sisi also penned a letter to her mother, stating, 'Both the emperor and I are shocked. There is no expression for his behaviour.'[38]

On the date that the wedding had been rescheduled, Ludwig wrote in his diary, 'Thanks be to God the fearful thing was not realised.'[39]

There is no record of why Ludwig had such a sudden change of heart that he could find no other way than to be cruel to such a sweet girl.

Less than two years passed, and Ludwig began dreaming of a new palace to build near the Linderhof. He wanted this one to have a formal garden built in Renaissance Style. He wanted it to emulate

Versailles and for it to be his refuge, where he could forget about the dreadful times in which he lived.

By May, plans were put in place for a lavish French palace surrounded by gardens, terraces, fountains, a sanctuary, a temple, and an artificial waterfall. He also designed an artificial cave with brilliant lights and coloured water. Ludwig watched his tribute to Louis XIV being built stone by stone. The building also served as an excuse for him to avoid court and the capital. He was so enthralled with the building that he forgot the fifth anniversary of the day he met Wagner, which he celebrated every year. He also forgot Wagner's birthday.

At the age of 24, Ludwig started to keep a diary, and it is a true confession of a man baring his soul to the world. He was a slave to himself and his repressed emotions. The more intolerant he became, the more suspicion – and even hatred – of the human race began to surface. His diary entries were often not dated; some were long, and some were short. Sometimes it was hard to tell where one began and the other left off.

He writes of how he indulges in sensual love and feels he has betrayed his idols. He says he is crying out for help to overcome what he feels is evil within him. Ludwig knew he was prone to violence, and Sisi had always been keen on his restlessness and instability during their relationship. At the time, mental specialists would recommend ice cold baths to reduce pathological excitability and unbearable headaches. Ludwig began to take carriage drives at night, and his physician found this to be very strange and sinister as he feared the moon may have taken control of his mental stability.

He repeatedly wrote about the royal bed in his diary, focusing on his admiration for Louis XIV. Was he perhaps enthralled with the French king's known sexual prowess and his endless supply of mistresses? He wrote of the mysticism of numbers and his obsession with the occult. He wrote of his brother Otto, who was also subjected to fits which were growing worse. Otto was always nervous and often didn't sleep for days on end. At one point, he wore the same pair of shoes for weeks, never taking them off. He spoke of how his brother would make odd faces and bark like a dog before becoming normal again. Otto's doctors had also begun to take notice of the prince's odd behaviour and compromised mental health.

When Wilhelm I was declared the new German emperor in January of 1871, Ludwig was very disappointed. He felt he should have been granted the honour and even threatened to abdicate in favour of his brother Otto.

In the summer of 1871, Ludwig acted out as if he were greeting groups of peasants and grooms in the forest for eating, drinking and horseplay.[40] This is very similar to Sisi's visions of visiting peasants for amusement. In October, the new Baden Diplomatic Envoy was granted an audience with the king and made several observations about him and his palace.

> The domestics were very queer. I know that the king lived very alone at Berg, except for a few servants. But there are no court officials and hardly any guards. The king was dressed in black and looked quite elegant. The bottom rooms of the palace were not very impressionable, with average furniture and artwork and an odd smell.[41]

Ludwig spent roughly three-quarters of a year at Hohenschwangau Castle, where he would read obsessively about Louis XIV in his many books on the French monarch. Ludwig rode out around midnight with his groomsman and once more wrote of Otto's health. But when we read his notes, he could have been speaking about himself: 'His nerves are in a state of irritability. He seldom dresses, hardly ever goes outside, like a wild animal, and has horrible hallucinations.'[42]

In March of 1873, the king met Baron Von Varicourt, a soldier from the Bavarian Army whom he made his personal assistant. As with his previous relationships, Ludwig fell for him immediately. His first letter to Varicourt speaks of his obsession with plays, French history, and Louis XIV. He also told him that he was the only one who deserved to sit next to him in the royal opera box and asked him to go to see a play.

Of his new position as personal assistant to the king, Varicourt replied, 'I am full of happiness about my new appointment.'[43]

In another letter to Varicourt, Ludwig says,

'I think with inmost joy of the hours which I had the pleasure of spending with you in the theatre and in the Winter Garden.'[44]

The king also made him promise not to talk to anyone about the things they discussed, especially politics. He wrote about his need for solitude and his dislike for most people. During one of their evenings together, Ludwig told his new friend how much he feared going to bed as he was plagued with terrible nightmares. They often would stay up late into the evening talking instead of sleeping.

While it's quite possible that Varicourt didn't share the same intensity for their relationship, in Ludwig's letters we again hear the desperation that radiated from his soul, and it causes us to sympathise with him. How unequivocally he seemed to find himself infatuated with someone new that it dominated his thoughts and time. It was as if he was always trying to establish intimacies when there was not much of a foundation:

> I am happy in the resemblance of the hours which I spent with you yesterday. But this feeling is mixed with sorrow because I had the impression that last night you were quite different from how you were the other day … the thought that you will always remember me in friendship would be a blessed consolation to me; the contrary would make me ill … the most beautiful and most longed for death for me would be to die for you. That death would be more desirable for me than anything else the world could offer.[45]

Varicourt seemed to have his own form of passion in the shape of a bad temper, and he often reacted to things crudely and violently, which undoubtedly caused Ludwig to fret even more: 'I ask for an explanation of this curious and completely incomprehensible phase. It would hurt me deeply if only the shadow of a doubt were to come between us.'[46]

But no matter how much Ludwig tried to bring Varicourt to the same level, it became clear that he wasn't interested in the same type of relationship. For Varicourt, when asked to become the king's personal assistant, we can imagine that the only answer accepted would have been yes. But with this position came the bizarre attachment Ludwig would soon form to his new attendant, and it's entirely understandable that Varicourt began to pull away if he began to feel uncomfortable. It is of the greatest honour to serve your sovereign, but what if that sovereign is a man who is slowly going mad?

As the consistency of Varicourt's letter began to thin, Ludwig was filled with deep loneliness and informed him that he was going to the mountains for a time. He saw Varicourt as more than a personal assistant. He was someone whom Ludwig felt had possessed the very depths of his soul. The second half of 1873 proved more miserable than Ludwig had ever experienced. Though his courtship with Varicourt was brief, it was intense, and as he slipped away, Ludwig felt more alone than ever.

His brother's mental health was also in a rapid decline and it seemed as if he would never recover. The family met at Hohenschwangau Castle for Ludwig's 28th birthday and it was there that Marie of Prussia may have finally come to realise that both of her sons were either insane or, at the least, very abnormal.

Dr Von Gudden (1824–1886) joined the family to discuss the latest reports on Otto's health and it was decided that he should be kept in Fürstenried Palace in Munich, which would become his domicile for years. Ludwig was too ashamed to visit his brother as he felt it might cause him to deteriorate further himself. He finally realised that he couldn't escape his own madness as he became more and more like his ill brother.

By June 1875 Otto seemed to worsen, and Ludwig wrote to his mother, 'Otto suffers more than ever from tormenting hallucinations and religious scruples.'[47]

In a September letter to Ludwig wrote to his prior governess, who had taken her married name, Frau Von Leonrod. They two had kept in touch since she was dismissed from his care in childhood. 'Pour Otto! For a long time, I had no news from him personally about his health. He seems to suffer more than we all imagined. He urgently needs a better doctor.'[48]

By the end of 1878, Otto was declared insane, and the king was utterly heartbroken.

The last seven years of Ludwig's life were the lowest, and he realised that he was slowly going mad, just as his brother had. His dislike for mankind and his feelings of loneliness only deepened. Between April and December 1879, he stayed in the mountains, only communicating through his devoted cabinet secretary Friedrich Von Zeigler. He claimed he wanted to leave Bavaria as it had become intolerable for him, but being the king, it was not a possibility.

By early 1881, the king's diary entries had become a rambling mess of incomplete sentences. One example was written after he dined in his Winter Garden with Wagner, and they spent some time together: 'was present with Richard Wagner at the performance of *Lohengrin*, very successful and beautiful. He presents, with him in the apartment in the Winter Garden, a long time together.'

He spoke of his memories of Marine Antionette before reverting to talk of Wagner: 'Cordial and sad. Happiness and blessing on his beloved head. Last fall, the double date of 18 (majority) and, by the greatest luck, another nearly one and a half years of twice the number of years of my life as 'King' 19 no more, no more, no more.'[49]

As it is clear to any reader, his words had become an incoherent cluster of nonsense.

In the spring of 1881, Ernst Von Possart, director of the Court Theatre (1841–1921), sent Ludwig a photograph of an Austrian actor by the name of Josef Kainz (1858–1920). He was 23 years old and had recently joined the Munich Court Theatre. His photo showed a boyish, wistful face with beautiful eyes and a sensitive mouth. Not surprisingly, the king was immediately smitten and ordered that Kainz play the part of Didier in a production of Hugo's *Marion de Lome*. Ludwig imagined himself as the Marquess de Sauverny and Kainz as Didier, the mysterious man who rescues her from her woes.

Ludwig was so impressed with the play that he sent Kainz a ring and a gold chain. He was convinced he was Didier and could think of him in no other way. He wrote in his diary: 'In the night arrived the actor of Didier.' He refused to use his real name, and in some bizarre twist of reality, Ludwig failed to see Kainz as a real person, giving him instead the fantasy persona of a character in a play. But when the king met Kainz in the flesh, underneath the costumes and vestments of the play, he was disappointed. He had nothing like the physique Ludwig had imagined him to have and instead was unimposing and small-framed.

Perhaps to chastise Kainz for not being what Ludwig imagined him to be, he forced him to read out of books for hours, with only Ludwig in attendance. As if this wasn't bizarre enough, if Kainz skipped a passage or misread a line incorrectly, the king immediately and harshly corrected him.

This is yet another example of how all of Ludwig's relationships were impulsive, causing him to act like a lovesick adolescent. He addressed many of his acquaintances as characters in a play much the same way he envisioned Marie Antoinette coming alive through his cousin Sisi. He continued living in a world caught between reality and his imagination of eccentric friendships.

Like many others before him, Kainz must have done something to upset the king because in a letter dated 16 June 1881, Kainz begs for Ludwig's forgiveness, saying: 'if I only knew by what I hurt Your Majesty so much!'

In February of 1883, Ludwig would suffer the devastating loss that he had written of so many times in his diary and letters. Richard Wagner, his beloved friend, died.

In the previous year, Wagner had become very ill, suffering from several several attacks of angina. He and Cosima travelled to Venice in early 1883 and suffered a heart attack that was apparently due to an argument between them. Cosima was so distraught over his death that at one point she threw herself over his coffin in misery.

Ludwig was grieving deeply too. Any feelings of resentment which had built up for Wagner over the years disappeared upon his death. A few days after the burial, he travelled to Bayreuth in Germany and stood by Wagner's grave throughout the night.

For Ludwig, Wagner had brought out the best in him when it came to dealing with other human beings. And yet, with everyone he met, his relationships ended in a quarrel, and he fell in love with people for who he wanted them to be, not who they actually were.

In 1884, Ludwig was visited by Dr Franz Karl, a 'mental' specialist, who was sent to see him for what was believed to be a toothache with the assumption that he could treat it, despite his specialty in psychiatric medicine. Ludwig told the doctor he was anxious about his eyes, and then began to ramble on incessantly for hours. Despite the oddness of this, Dr Karl was so taken by how well-spoken the king was that he said there couldn't possibly be anything wrong with his brain.

During the last few months of Ludwig II's life, he refused to even look at his servants. He took to writing them notes on scraps of paper. Sometimes these notes lay where the servants may find them easily, and other times, the king simply shoved the paper underneath their doors. If a servant needed to visit Ludwig for any reason, they were instructed to make a scratching noise at the door. They needed to remain in a bow once admitted and not look at His Majesty under any circumstances.

One of the odd notes left by Ludwig, dated 13 December 1885 read: 'Cutlets, beer. Ham bad, the latter cooked badly. When I come back from Mass, one bottle of champagne, one dish foie gras, and five hundred marks.'[50]

The king also demanded that his pencils be sharpened without having to ask, and that his coffee must never come to him boiling hot as he would drink it only after one hour. He wrote another berating note to a servant on 20 December, stating it was a scandal that his servant didn't tie his tie correctly, and that he always had to fix it. In writing about a desired teapot the following days, he said:

> It must be Chinese and not Japanese. The blue must be purer and more radiating as on the vase. The cups are to be big and round. The upper edges to be very broad and all in gold with relief work only, and the blue is to begin on the blue ground, all to be the gold relief figures from China. Buildings, landscapes, birds, and dragons.[51]

In January 1886, we read perhaps one of the most heartbreaking diary entries thus far: 'God, give me the power so that I may conquer the evil, subdue the senses, so that not once can there be any question in this book of a relapse.' Then quoting the flamboyant poet, Lord Byron, he writes, 'I am thus wasting the best part of my life, daily repenting and never amending.'[52]

It became harder and harder for servants to gain access to the king, so the army sent selected private soldiers instead. Most of Ludwig's servants disliked the solitude of the palace and didn't know how to deal with his strange and unpredictable personality. He soon demanded that all letters be directly written to his private secretary, Richard Hornig. He spoke of the hurray to finish his throne room at Residenz Palace and his bedroom at Linderhof. He also demanded that Neuschwanstein Castle be completed by 1889. While a painting of Louis XIV was already on the ceiling in the Residenz Palace, he insisted on additional artwork in other rooms. He had pictures from the *Tannhäuser Saga*, episodes of *Tristan and Isolde*, along with paintings of the Blessed Mother and the Ascension of Christ. In his sitting room, he wanted representations from *Saga of the Knights of the Swan*.

In the king's Schloss Berg castle, there was excessive use of the colour blue, the walls were blue with gold fleurs de lis, and there were gold stars on the ceiling. The curtains and upholstery were blue with extensive fringing. Busts of his father and grandfather, as well as Wagner, stood on marble pedestals. A statue of Lohengrin drawing his sword and one of Tell with his bow dominated the room. The walls were adorned with paintings of Wanger's operas. His sitting room, bedroom and dining rooms had hideous metal gas chandeliers hanging from the ceiling.

Oddly enough, the gatehouse may have been the only place the king stayed for any length of time. It was complete with a winding stone staircase, a living room in simple Bavarian décor, and two small bedrooms with mattresses covered with red Turkey cotton. It was here that he could stay to watch the construction of his buildings take place and talk to the workers. The only problem was that he was micromanaging all the ministers of the building.

Hornig was, however, very devoted to Ludwig, always showing dignity and self-composure and never participating in gossip. He had an incredible amount of patience with the king. In one incident when the two were out riding, Hornig was forced to dismount his horse several times to adjust the king's riding gear. Hornig often returned from these outings utterly exhausted. Ludwig also sent him all over Europe, dealing with architects and giving reports about other buildings. He knew the king could be very cruel and fly into a rage over the smallest things.

When staying at Schloss Chiemsee, Ludwig would walk up and down the mirrored hallway that emulated Versailles from 9 pm to 6 am, discussing plans for future castles to be constructed. He would instruct Hornig to stand absolutely still for the entire day, over twelve hours. This exhausting ritual was a rigid German tradition among royals – including Queen Victoria.

On its southern side, Neuschwanstein Castle rises directly up from a rocky gorge 300 ft deep at the bed of the River Pollatt. The gorge is spanned by a narrow suspension bridge made of steel cables. Ludwig once ordered Hornig to ride across the bridge on horseback, watching in delight as he and his horse swung from side to side.

One could not expect that anyone would endure the humiliation that Hornig put up with for very long. And one day in May of 1867, he'd finally had enough. He hated seeing a group of dirty, lazy soldiers taking over, and he thought Ludwig's treatment of his servants was cruel. He had witnessed the king throwing things at them, and he made them crawl to him on their bellies before he would purposely hit them. Hornig said he could no longer be the king's secretary, which caused him to fly into a rage, ordering Hornig to leave the castle and never return.

The king's scrawls on pieces of paper continued and became almost unreadable and more bizarre. In one note, we see the king writing of a servant called Hiedl, whom he liked because of the sound of his voice. He instructed him to 'rub oil on his neck to keep it warm and take care of himself. I want to know, what are his manners, what age is he?'[53] He also instructed another servant that he was not to grow a moustache. And yet other servants were continuously sent away and denied fresh water for washing. His notes and demands became brasher.

'The door to the balcony is always to be shut when I have passed it. Again, left undone. Write it down!'

He made ridiculous demands about the temperature in the castle and suddenly changed the time his supper was to be delivered. In his diary, he complained about the soldiers doing his bidding, 'They do nothing but give bad service. Horrible pants, too; both buttons have gone.' and then changed the subject to something totally irrelevant, such as 'Beautiful flowers need to be sent to Archduchess Elisabeth, and then immediately back to how he had bad milk and that someone needed to investigate for vermin. Another of his demanding notes to his servants was scolding them when his vegetables weren't brought to him on time.

When he wrote to his mother, he told her about a toothache but denied her a visit as he didn't want her to see him in such a state of melancholy. He told her of a hallucination where he had pulled his dead father from his coffin and boxed his ears. On top of his complicated mental status, the king also suffered from horrific headaches and had very little sleep. For this, he took chloral and soporifics several times a day and often had ice applied to his head.

By June 1886, the Bavarian Government was building a case to force Ludwig to abdicate. He had neglected his royal duties and spent ridiculous amounts of money on Wagner and his operas, as well as building three unnecessary castles with plans in place for a fourth. As there no provision made to keep Otto from the succession, he would naturally become king should Ludwig be removed – effectively replacing one 'lunatic' king with another. However, there was a clause in the constitution stating that if a sovereign became unable to perform his duties, a regency could be provided. It was under this clause that the government and the king's uncle, Prince Luitpold (1821–1912,) built their case; after Otto, Prince Luitpold was the nearest male relative to inherit the throne. However, as half of the elective power lay with the king it was essentially one half of the constitution against the other. Consequently, Otto would have been next in line to the throne but it would have been quite the job to rule both brother's insane, but what choice did they have? On 1 June 1886, Prince Luitpold penned a letter to the Ministerial Counsellor, Dr Von Zeigler:

> The obvious illness of His Majesty The King has, as you know, put the country in a very sad predicament so that I consider it my duty to consider taking measures which, within the constitution, would guarantee the continuity of the government. For this purpose, it is absolutely necessary to get as exact a picture as possible of the mental state of His Majesty The King.

Meetings and reports were gathered from the king's personal groom, Hesselschwerdt, and Welcker, his footman. Four of Ludwig's doctors agreed that a physical exam was not necessary and Dr Von Gudden signed off on a report that became the basis for further action to remove him from the throne.

The king got wind of what was happening from his coachman, and he summoned the police and fire brigade, as well as village peasants who supported him. They all responded in his favour. When the delegation team came to the castle's gatehouse to seize the king, they were met by an angry crowd of his supporters, bearing rifles, axes, and scythes. The officer guarding the gatehouse said anyone who tried to enter would be shot. In an absolute rage, Ludwig threatened to have the delegation team beheaded, causing them to retreat.

The Bavarian government feared a civil war was on their hands as Ludwig drew up a proclamation claiming the actions of the committee to have him removed was treason. Somehow, this document written by the king was confiscated, and he was eventually taken prisoner at Berg. Dr Von Gudden and other psychiatrists gave orders to have his apartments turned into a prison, where he would be alone except for a few frightened servants. Ludwig spent the night of 10 June wandering from room to room, escaping into his own fantasy world. He began speaking aloud to several dead spirits, including Marie Antoinette and Louis XIV. The king was mentally incapacitated, penniless, and without any hope. His uncle Luitpold took over the rule of the kingdom and acted as regent in Ludwig's place.

The following day, a team of doctors, mental specialists, police, and one of Ludwig's prior servants came to the castle, where his valet admitted them as he was afraid that Ludwig was on the verge of suicide. Earlier in the day, Ludwig had repeatedly demanded the key to the castle's tower, which was 200 ft high and would have easily been the end for Ludwig had he jumped. Dr Von Gudden and the others were armed with a straightjacket when Ludwig was finally given the tower key. He immediately headed for the staircase, so it seemed certain that he planned to end his life by throwing himself from the tower. He was restrained by two doctors, and the straightjacket was placed on him. Following a seizure, Ludwig composed himself but continued to question Dr Von Gudden: 'Without examining me, how can you pronounce the state of my health?'[54]

Von Gudden continued to assure him that an exam was not necessary. Spies had already gone through his waste baskets at his previous living quarters and found crumpled diary entries and his obscure notes. After several hours, Ludwig finally agreed to accompany Dr Von Gudden. In the early hours of 12 June, Ludwig stepped into a waiting coach. A nurse was sitting next to the driver, and the handles of the coach's doors were altered so Ludwig could not escape. While the rest of the entourage was able to stop to relieve themselves and freshen up at roadside inns, the king was given a rudely constructed commode and not given any food for almost fifteen hours.

When they arrived at Berg, he was finally given something to eat and put to bed. It was said that he talked in his sleep all night. Builders were sent to Berg the next day to configure putting bars on the windows, and the noise from all the banging drove Ludwig into a frenzy of anxiety. He was granted an audience with his doctors and remained courteous as he asked to hear Mass; his request was denied.

That evening, after dinner, Ludwig and Dr Von Gudden went for a walk with no servants or police in attendance. They hadn't returned when promised, and a police officer was sent to look for them. Several hours into his search, the king's hat, jacket, overcoat, and umbrella were found on the shore of a lake. More people were called in, and a steward then discovered two bodies lying a short distance apart. While Von Gudden's feet were still on dry ground, his face was in the water as if he had been held underwater. The king's body lay only a few feet away in the shallow water. They were both pulled to shore, and attempts were made to save them, but to no avail. Both Dr Von Gudden and King Ludwig II had perished.

They were taken back to the palace and laid out in separate bedrooms. Doctors were called to examine them. Von Gudden's face was badly scratched, and his right eye was bruised. He was also missing a fingernail. One doctor claimed he saw strangulation marks on his neck, but this was never confirmed. When the king was examined, there was not a mark on his face.

When hearing the news, Prince Luitpold burst into tears at the death of his nephew. Empress Elisabeth sent a bouquet of flowers to be placed in the king's hands. The Bavarian people were devastated by the death of their king, and rumours began to circulate that he had been murdered. But his autopsy showed nothing out of the ordinary, and his cause of death was undetermined.

Dressed in the robes of the Grand Master of the Knights, Ludwig lay in state, covered with the ermine robe of state, surrounded by flowers and candles. He was buried in the noble court church of St Michael's, among several other members of the Wittelsbach family.

Speculation about the king's death is that he did, in fact, commit suicide as feared by his valet. Is it possible that he simply removed his coat and hat and tried to drown himself, with Von Gudden trying to intervene? Did Ludwig fight him off to the point of death before killing himself? Investigators suggested that there were footsteps and signs of a struggle on the shore of the lake, indicating some sort of foul play.

Today King Ludwig II is remembered as an eccentric monarch riddled with mental illness. No one will know for sure what lurked behind those deep blues eyes, but there was certainly some mystery regarding Ludwig's troubled thoughts. We must give him credit for being unbothered by his blatant homosexuality. The nineteenth century would not have been kind to anyone who preferred their own sex, never mind a monarch. And yet Ludwig openly expressed his love of men without much thought, which at least shows strength of character in his longing to put love first. For a man destined to be a king, his passion for the arts and for falling in love makes him stand out among many.

* * * *

Upon the death of Ludwig, his brother Otto became King Otto I – the king who never reigned; although he officially sat on the throne, his uncle, Prince Luitpold, ruled as regent. As we know by this time, Otto had already been declared legally insane and was mentally unfit to rule.

Otto was born on 27 April 1848, a little less than three years after his brother, and as we know, the brothers spent much of their childhood together at Hohenschwangau Castle. While his brother was more reclusive, Otto was rather outgoing and friendly in his younger years. In 1848, when he was 15, he started his brief career in the Bavarian Army. By his 18th birthday, he was promoted to captain. When King Maximilian II died, and Ludwig inherited the crown, Otto's responsibilities increased too. The brothers remained close and performed many royal duties at each other's side.

Around the time of the Franco-Prussian War in 1870, the darkness of mental illness began to surround Otto, and he grew depressed. Filled with anxiety, Otto began to tread the same path as his brother, avoiding people and seeking more and more time to be alone. This worried his family greatly. Otto seemed to go through spells where he would sleep poorly for days and act irrationally, followed by periods of total lucidity. His illness continued to worsen, as we've learned through Ludwig's letters. By the time he was declared insane in 1872, plans were already in place for what to do with him, including him spending much of his life shut away.

Starting in 1873, he was kept in isolation in the southern pavilion of Nymphenburg Palace, where he was attended by Dr Von Gudden. He was then moved to Schleissheim Palace, where it seems he was heavily drugged by Dr Von Gudden. It may or may not have been an attempt to treat him, as the treatment for mental illness was still in its primitive stages at the time.

His condition continued to worsen, and in 1883, he was sent to Fürstenried Palace, where he was kept under close medical supervision, and where he would remain for the rest of his life. He was visited by his brother on several occasions, and it was ordered that no violence ever be inflicted upon him.

In 1886, a statement written by the senior medical officer declared that Otto might have been suffering from schizophrenia. This is the same year that Otto became king of Bavaria upon Ludwig's death as per Wittelsbach law. Otto didn't understand that he had inherited the throne when it was explained to him. He believed his Uncle Luitpold was the real king, even after Bavarian troops were sworn in in his name and coins were manufactured with his image.

King Otto died in 1916 from an obstruction of the bowel.

Because he never truly reigned, Otto I is easily forgotten in Bavarian history, especially since he was overshadowed by his brother. And so, much like his brother, he spent the majority of his life struggling with the demons of his mental illness.

It is surely no secret that the Wittelsbach dynasty had its share of mental disturbances, most likely caused by the repeated inter-royal marriage throughout the family. And aside from Sisi, Ludwig and his brother Otto, there were other blood relatives who suffered throughout their lives.

Princess Alexandra of Bavaria (1826–1875), Ludwig's paternal aunt, is also known for her psychological issues. Alexandra never married as her father refused to allow anyone to take her hand in marriage because her health was too delicate. Instead, she lived her life as a talented writer, publishing several books of stories in both German and French. She also had an interest in children's theatre and devoted her life to the arts. In this way, she is very much like her nephew, King Ludwig, as the two shared a passion for such things.

Sadly, like both her nephews, Alexandra was plagued throughout her life with several mental issues. She was an easily agitated young lady with a liking for cleanliness that can easily be compared to some form of obsessive-compulsive disorder. She was so obsessed with cleanliness that she only wore white clothing. As a young adult, Alexandra developed a psychiatric disorder in which she believed she had swallowed a glass piano that could easily shatter within her at any moment. The beautiful princess with the mouse-brown hair and soft baby-blue eyes, was known to walk gingerly through the corridors of her home, turning awkwardly to fit through doors and avoiding any contact with any object that would destroy her glass instrument.

The delusion of being made of glass was not a new one and seemed to be a common affliction from the Middle Ages. An essay written by Gill Speak in the *History of Psychiatry* states that:

> The fear of being too fragile for this world was believed to be especially common among the nobility, as well as educated men, who may have read medical accounts of the delusion before ending up developing the symptoms themselves.

In a previous chapter, we learned that this same illness also affected King Charles VI of France. He believed that he was made of glass and had a suit of iron ribs made to protect him from any person or object around him.

The condition became so well known that in 1612, Robert Burton wrote of it in his *'Anatomy of Melancholy'* in 1612: 'Fear of devils, death, that they shall be so sick, of some such or such disease, ready to tremble at every object ... that they are all glass, and therefore will suffer no man to come near them.'

When Alexandra died on 21 September 1875, King Ludwig said of her death: 'Although it is always painful for the survivors when a member leaves the family circle forever, it really was a very good thing in the case of dear Aunt Alexandria. Her continuous sufferings from her nervous disease were seldom interrupted by moments of happiness.'[55]

The same perils of mental illness struck the uncle of Ludwig's mother. Frederick William (1795–1861), who became king of Prussia in 1840, reigned during the 1848 German Revolution, converting Prussia into a constitutional monarchy. After the revolution, King Frederick, much like King Ludwig, began withdrawing from the public eye. In May of 1848, Dr Jacobi, leading physician at the

Rhenish Lunatic Asylum at Siegburg, was called to the king, who was believed to be suffering from inflammation of the brain and a 'rattled nervous system'.

In 1855, during a visit to the Rhine at Cologne, Frederick appeared as a mere shadow of his former self, with shrunken eyes that swirled with restless anxiety. He seemed to suffer terribly when speaking, stumbling over his words, and losing the thread of the sentence he was trying to form.

His queen, Elisabeth Ludovika of Bavaria (1801-1873), as all too aware of her husband's struggles. Perhaps she exhibited a comforting nature to him, as the king soon would have no audience with anyone except her. He went nowhere without her, and the two became inseparable as his illness developed. He was reported to have physical scuffles involving his ministers that often resulted in bodily injuries to both.

To avoid public attention to his behaviour, King Frederick was reported to have suffered from dropsy, a term used for any swelling or oedema. His Majesty was seen having several small accidents, such as catching his face on a tree branch or falling over a stone and bumping his leg, and these incidents began to increase in frequency. In what seemed to be bouts of insanity, the king suddenly thought he was just a non-commissioned officer in the army. Despite his decline, like Ludwig, Fredrick William IV was kept on the throne. Through his mental illness, among quarrels with staff and members of the royal family, doctors said he suffered from such 'softening of the brain' that it was feared he might die.

The queen took advantage of his moments of lucidity, trying to make him aware of the Prussian people and to interact with the public, reminding him that he was king. Upon attending the wedding of the queen of Portugal, King Fredrick believed he was the bridegroom and was said to have made some 'odd remarks'. Another time, during a traditional dinner with some of the area's fishermen, the king suddenly rose from his seat, demanding that he be put in a frying pan.

On 24 November 1859, King Fredrick of Prussia suffered a stroke that forced him to spend the rest of his life in a wheelchair. He suffered another stroke a year later, and in January of 1861, another stroke caused his death.

It's hard to say whether these strokes had anything to do with the king's mental illness, but they must have further altered his mental state.

The throne would pass to his brother, Wilhelm I, who had become his regent in 1858. Wilhelm was the first head of state of a united Germany.

The Wittelsbachs would reign as kings of Bavaria until the Second World War. In 1921, Prince Rupprecht became head of the family, and earned Hitler's hatred by being in opposition to the Beer Hall Putsch in 1923. As he continued to voice his resistance against the Nazis, Rupprecht went into exile in Italy in 1939. Several members of his family were detained and forced into Nazi concentration camps.

After the war, Rupprecht returned to Munich and lived at his childhood home, Schloss Leutstetten, where he died in 1955.

The Wittelsbach empire is remembered as the dynasty that ruled and moulded Bavaria. Still, like many of the European empires, it is also remembered for the cluster of rulers that suffered from genetic abnormalities. These afflictions that spanned decades through Europe's royal families haunted some of the most powerful people this world has known.

* * * *

From Cleopatra in the Ancient Egyptian empire to the European Monarchies of the recent past, there have been triumphs and failures that were compromised simply by the genetic hands they were dealt. And still, for the most part, they persevered.

Work Cited

Chapter Four

1. Rushton, Alan, Royal Maladies Inherited Diseases in the Ruling Houses of Europe (Tafford Publishing 2008) p.83
2. Ibid p 84
3. ibid
4. ibid
5. R.C. Famiglietti, Royal Intrigue: Crisis at the Court of Charles VI, 1986 p.86-88
6. ibid
7. Rushton, Alan, Royal Maladies Inherited Diseases in the Ruling Houses of Europe (Tafford Publishing 2008) p.84
8. ibid p.79
9. ibid
10. ibid
11. Johnson, Lauren, History Today, The Madness of King Henry VI 2019
12. Rushton, Alan, Royal Maladies Inherited Diseases in the Ruling Houses of Europe (Tafford Publishing 2008) p.70
13. Great Books Guy, The Plantagenants, 2021
14. Rushton, Alan, Royal Maladies Inherited Diseases in the Ruling Houses of Europe (Tafford Publishing 2008) p.80

Chapter Five

1. Fox, Julia, Sister Queens, Ballantine Books 2011 p.101
2. ibid

3. ibid
4. Fox, Julia, Sister Queens, Ballantine Books 2011 p.125
5. ibid p.131
6. ibid p.137
7. ibid
8. ibid p.205
9. ibid p.210
10. ibid p.226
11. ibid p.224
12. ibid p.252
13. ibid p.254

Chapter Six

1. Rushton, Alan, Royal Maladies Inherited Diseases in the Ruling Houses of Europe (Tafford Publishing 2008) p.70
2. ibid p.69
3. ibid
4. ibid p.70
5. ibid p.68
6. ibid

Chapter Seven

1. The Creative Historian, On This Day: Birth of Sophia Dorothea of Celle, 2016
2. Rushton, Alan, Royal Maladies Inherited Diseases in the Ruling Houses of Europe (Tafford Publishing 2008) p.51
3. Ibid
4. ibid p.41
5. ibid
6. Hibbert, Christopher, George III (Basic Books) 1998 p.258
7. Ibid p.259

8. ibid
9. ibid p.260
10. Ibid p.261
11. ibid
12. ibid
13. ibid p.278
14. ibid p.286
15. ibid p.289
16. ibid p.315
17. ibid p.316
18. ibid
19. ibid p.318
20. Ibid p.340
21. Ibid p.343
22. ibid p.394

Chapter Eight

1. Potts, D.M, Victoria's Gene: Haemophilia and the Royal Family Sutton Publishing 1999 p. 3
2. ibid
3. ibid p.5
4. ibid p.6
5. ibid p.7
6. ibid p.29
7. ibid p.30
8. ibid p.37
9. ibid p.39
10. ibid p.37
11. ibid p.38
12. ibid p.39
13. ibid p.40
14. ibid

15. ibid p.41
16. ibid p.41
17. ibid p.42
18. ibid
19. ibid
20. ibid p.51

Chapter Nine

1. Bloks, Moniek, Tsaravich Alexei: The Boy With Haemophilia 2018
2. Massie, Robert, Nicholas and Alexandra 1967 p.137

Chapter Ten

1. O'Malley, Charles, Some Episodes in the Medical History of Emperor Charles V, Stanford University, 1965 p.470
2. ibid
3. ibid p.472
4. ibid p.474
5. ibid
6. Langdon-Davies, John, Carlos The King Who Would Not Die, Johnathan Cape LTD, 1962 p.51
7. ibid
8. ibid p.91
9. ibid p.96
10. ibid p.122
11. ibid p.124
12. ibid p.125
13. ibid
14. ibid p.168
15. ibid
16. ibid p.187
17. ibid p.201

18. ibid
19. ibid p.238
20. Bohn, Henry, History of the House of Austria from 1218 to 1792, London p. 515
21. Wheatcroft, Andrew, The Habsburgs: Embodying Empire, Penguin p.249

Chapter Eleven

1. Chauviere, Emily, The Marriage of Emperor Francis Joseph and Elisabeth of Austria 2011
2. Tschudi, Clara, Elisabeth Empress of Austria and Queen of Hungary E.P. Dutton 1901 p.59
3. Ibid p. 71
4. ibid p.90
5. Ibid p.135
6. ibid p.224
7. ibid p.226
8. ibid
9. Ibid p 232
10. ibid p.238
11. ibid p.239
12. ibid p.243
13. ibid p.245
14. ibid p.248
15. Chaptman-Huston, Desmond, Ludwig II The Mad King of Bavaria Dorset Press 1900 p.23
16. ibid p.31
17. ibid p.38
18. ibid p.39
19. ibid p.46
20. ibid p. 49
21. ibid p.58

22. ibid
23. ibid p.67
24. Ibid p.75
25. Ibid p. 80
26. Ibid p.81
27. Ibid p.76
28. Ibid p.84
29. Ibid p.85
30. Ibid p.93
31. Ibid
32. Ibid p.100
33. Ibid p.106
34. Ibid p.121
35. Ibid p.122
36. Ibid p.124
37. Ibid p.135
38. Ibid p.137
39. Ibid
40. Ibid p.170
41. Ibid p.171
42. Ibid p.176
43. Ibid p.182
44. Ibid
45. Ibid p.186
46. Ibid p.188
47. Ibid p.202
48. Ibid p.208
49. Ibid p.216
50. Ibid p.251
51. Ibid p.253
52. Ibid
53. Ibid p.262
54. Ibid p.285
55. Ibid p.201

Bibliography

Abrams, H. (2006). *Gregor Mendel: Planting the Seeds of Genetics.* Simon Mawer.

Ashley, M. (1965). *Louis XIV and the Greatness of France.* Free Press.

Ashton, J. (2006). *Unwrapping the Pharaoh.* Master Books.

Barlag, P. (2021). *Evil Roman Emperors: The Shocking History of Ancient Rome's Most Wicked Rulers from Caligula to Nero and More.* Prometheus.

Bessel, R. (1993). *Germany After the First War.* Clarendon Press.

Bloks, M. (2018). Tsaravich Alexei: The Boy With Haemophilia.

Bohn, H. (n.d.). *History of the House of Austria from 1218 to 1792.* London.

Breverton, T. (2019). *Henry VII: The Maligned Tudor King.* Amberley Publishing.

Carter, H. (2013). *Discovering Tutankhamen: From Howard Carter to DNA.* American University in Cairo Press.

Chaptman-Huston, D. (1900). *Ludwig II The Mad King of Bavaria.* Dorset Press.

Chauviere, E. (2011). *The Marriage of Emperor Francis Joseph and Elisabeth of Austria.*

Cost, B. (2023). Meet the Whittakers. *New York Post.*

Craig, W. (2017). *Memoir of Her Majesty Sophia Charlotte Mecklenburg Strelitz.* Creative Media Partners.

Deady, K. (2011). *Ancient Egypt.* Capstone.

Dean, G. (1971). *The Porphyrias A Story of Inheritance and Enviroment.* Pitman Medical.

Faris, D. (2007). The Fugate Family of Russell County. Gateway Press.

Firestone, G. (2012). *Rasputi and Alexei The Last Romanov.* America Star Books.

Fox, J. (2011). *Sister Queens.* Ballantine Books.

Fraser, A. (1979). *Royal Charles: Charles II and the Restoration.* Knopf.

Gaskoin, C. (2108). *History of the House of Hanover.* Ozymandias Press.

Goldberg, H. (2017). *Hippocrates, Father of Medicine.* Muriwai Books.

Green, D. (2014). *The Hundred Years War A People's History.* Yale University Press.

Guy, G. B. (2002). The Plantagenants.

Hazen, C. (2021). *The History of the Napoleonic Wars.* Art Now.

Henneberger, M. (1993). Adirondack Hamlet Defies Time. *New York Times.*

Hibbert, C. (1998). *George III.* Basic Books.

Hill, D. (1012). *The Royal Family: A Year by Year Chronicle of the House of Windsor.* Parragon Book.

Historian, T. C. (2016). On This Day; The Birth of Sophia Dorothea of Celle.

Janzen, R. (2010). *The Hurrerites in North America.* John Hopkins University Press.

Johnson, L. (2020). *Shadow King: The Life and Death of Henry VI.* Head of Zeus.

Jones, D. (2013). *The Plantagenets: The Warrior Kings and Queens Who Made England.* Penguin.

Katira, V. (2017). *Basics of Human Genetics.* CBS Publishers.

Knecht, R. (2007). *The Valois Kings of France 1328-1589.* Bloomsbury Academic.

Kokkonen, A. (2022). *The Politics of Succession.* OUP Oxford.

Langdon-Davies, J. (1962). *Carlos: The King Who Would Not Die.* Jonathan Cape LTD.

233

Lever, E. (2001). *Marie Antoinette: The Last Queen of France.* St. Martins Publishing Group.

Lewis, J. (1998). *Mary Queen of Scots Romance and Nation.* Routledge.

Lynch, J. (2103). *The Medieval Church.* Taylor & Francis.

Massie, R. (1967). *Nicholas and Alexandra.*

Mayhew, M. (2023). *Rasputinand His Russian Queen.* Pen & Sword.

McKendrick, M. (2105). *Ferdinand and Isabella.* New World City.

McMeekin, S. (2017). *The Russian Revolution: A New History.* Basic Books.

McQuillan, R. (2009). *Homozygosity, Inbreeding and Health in European Populations.* University of Ediburgh.

Meyer, G. J. (2011). *The Tudors: The Complete Story of England's Most Notorious Dynasty.* Random House.

New Zealand Origin Incest Colt Clan. (2021). *New Zealand Herald.*

O'Malley, C. (1965). *Some Episodes in the Medical History of Emperor Charles V.* Standford University.

Parker, G. (2019). *Emperor: A New Life of Charles V.* Yale University Press.

Porter, L. (2010). *Mary Tudor: The First Queen.* Little, Brown Book Group.

Potts, D. (1999). *Victoria's Gene: Haemophilia and the Royal Family.* Sutton Publishing.

Quammen, D. (2007). *The Reluctant Mr. Darwin.* W.W. Norton.

Ramiglietti, R. (1986). *Royal Intrigue: Crisis at the Court of Charles VI.*

River, C. (2017). *The Ptolemaic Kingdom.* CreatSpace.

Rushton, A. (2008). *Royal Maladies Inherited Diseases in the Rules Houses of Europ.* Tafford Publishing.

Siraisi, N. (2009). *Medieval and Early Renaissance Medicine.* University of Chicago Press.

Steane, J. (2003). *The Archaeology of the Medieval Monarchy.* Taylor and Francis.

Thoneman, P. (2106). *The Hellenistic Age.* Oxford University.

Tschudi, C. (1901). *Elisabeth Empress of Austria and Queen of Hungary.* E.P Dutton.

Van der Kiste, J. (2011). *Queen Victoria's Children.* History Press.

Watkins, S.-B. (2017). *Margaret Tudor, Queen of Scots.* John Hunt Publishing Limited.

Weir, A. (2012). *Eleanor of Aquitaine.* Random House.

Wheatcroft, A. (n.d.). *The Habsburgs: Embodying Empire.* Penguin.